Clinician's Endodontic Handbook

Clinician's Endodontic Handbook

Thom C. Dumsha, MS, DDS, MS
Associate Professor and Chair
Department of Endodontics
University of Maryland Baltimore College of Dental Surgery
Dental School
University of Maryland
Baltimore, Maryland

James L. Gutmann, DDS, FACD, FICD
Professor and Director of Graduate Endodontics
The Texas A & M University System
Health Science Center
Baylor College of Dentistry
Dallas, Texas

LEXI-COMP INC
Hudson (Cleveland)

NOTICE

This handbook is intended to serve the user as a handy quick reference and not as a complete reference resource. While great care has been taken to ensure the accuracy of the information presented, the reader is advised that the authors, editors, reviewers, contributors, and publishers cannot be responsible for the continued currency of the information or for any errors, omissions, or the application of this information, or for any consequences arising therefrom. Therefore, the author(s) and/or the publisher shall have no liability to any person or entity with regard to claims, loss, or damage caused, or alleged to be caused, directly or indirectly, by the use of information contained herein. Because of the dynamic nature of drug information, readers are advised that decisions regarding drug therapy must be based on the independent judgment of the clinician, changing information about a drug (eg, as reflected in the literature and manufacturer's most current product (information), and changing medical practices. The editors are not responsible for any inaccuracy of quotation or for any false or misleading implication that may arise due to the text or formulas as used or due to the quotation of revisions no longer official.

The editors, authors, and contributors have written this book in their private capacities. No official support or endorsement by any federal agency or pharmaceutical company is intended or inferred.

The publishers have made every effort to trace the copyright holders for borrowed material. If they have inadvertently overlooked any, they will be pleased to make the necessary arrangements at the first opportunity.

If you have any suggestions or questions regarding any information presented in this handbook, please contact Lexi-Comp at

1-877-837-LEXI (5394)

This manual was produced using the FormuLex™ Program — a complete publishing service of Lexi-Comp Inc.

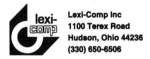

lexi-comp

Lexi-Comp Inc
1100 Terex Road
Hudson, Ohio 44236
(330) 650-6506

ISBN 0-916589-95-1

TABLE OF CONTENTS

ABOUT THE AUTHORS

Thom C. Dumsha, MS, DDS, MS

Dr Thom Dumsha is Associate Professor and Chair of the Department of Endodontics, University of Maryland at Baltimore College of Dental Surgery. Dr Dumsha graduated from the University of Maryland Dental School where he also received his certificate in Endodontics. He has earned a Master of Science Degree in Physiology from the Graduate School at the University of Maryland Baltimore and a Master of Science Degree in Information Systems from the University of Maryland Baltimore County. He is a Diplomate of the American Board of Endodontics.

Dr Dumsha served as the Program Director for the Advanced Specialty Program in Endodontics at the University of Maryland for 10 years. He has been an active member of the AAE, ADA, AADS, AADR, and IADR. He has received multiple teaching awards including the Frank J. Sinnreich, Jr Award for Excellence in Teaching, the Alpha Omega Clinical Teaching Award, and the Russell Gigliotti Memorial Award.

Dr Dumsha has published numerous articles particularly in his field of expertise dealing with dental trauma. He is coauthor of the *Problem Solving in Endodontics* textbook that is currently in its third edition and has been printed in four languages. Dr Dumsha lectures both nationally and internationally. Although a full-time faculty member at the University, he also maintains a part-time endodontic practice. Because of his background and degree in Information Systems, Dr Dumsha is also responsible for setting up and maintaining the server-based NT digital radiography system in the Department of Endodontics.

James L. Gutmann, DDS, FACD, FICD

A native of Wisconsin, Dr James L. Gutmann received his DDS. in 1970 from Marquette University School of Dentistry and his Certificate of Advanced Specialty Training in Endodontics from the University of Illinois College of Dentistry. After serving two years in the military at Ft Lee Virginia, he spent one year in full-time private endodontic practice in Springfield Massachusetts. He entered academia as an Assistant Professor of Endodontics at the Medical College of Virginia in 1975. In 1976, he was appointed as Chairman of the Department of Endodontics at the Baltimore College of Dental Surgery, University of Maryland at Baltimore. In 1982, Dr Gutmann was appointed as a tenured Professor and Chairman of the Department of Endodontics at Baylor College of Dentistry in Dallas Texas.

Presently he is Professor and Director of the Graduate Endodontic Program within the Department of Restorative Sciences at Baylor. Dr Gutmann is a Diplomate of the American Board of Endodontics, a member of the Scientific Advisory Panel of the *Journal of Endodontics* and the *Arab Dental Journal*, Editorial Board of the *Journal of the History of Dentistry*, and an Associate Editor of the *International Endodontic Journal*. He is a member of the Executive Committee of the American Association of Endo-dontists, serving as its President-Elect and he will become the 57th President of the AAE in 2000. He has presented over 500 lectures, papers, and continuing education courses in the United States and 33 foreign countries on six continents. Additionally he has authored or coauthored over 150 articles in both dental journals and texts that address scientific, research, educational, and clinical topics. He is the senior author of an endodontic text entitled *Problem Solving in Endodontics* published in its third edition in 1997. He is also the senior coauthor of the text entitled *Surgical Endodontics*, published in 1991 and reprinted in 1994 and 1998. In 1998, he was awarded an honorary doctorate from the University of Athens, Athens Greece for his contributions to dentistry and endodontics. In 2000, he will be honored as the Alumnus of the Year – Marquette University School of Dentistry.

EDITORIAL ADVISORY PANEL

David S. Jacobs, MD
President, Pathologists Chartered
Overland Park, Kansas

Bernard L. Kasten, Jr, MD
Vice-President/Medical Director
Corning Clinical Laboratories
Teteroboro, New Jersey

Polly E. Kintzel, PharmD
Clinical Pharmacy Specialist
Bone Marrow Transplantation, Detroit Medical Center
Harper Hospital
Detroit, Michigan

Donna M. Kraus, PharmD
Associate Professor of Pharmacy Practice
Departments of Pharmacy Practice and Pediatrics
Pediatric Clinical Pharmacist
University of Illinois at Chicago
Chicago, Illinois

Charles Lacy, PharmD, FCSHP
Clinical Coordinator and Drug Information Specialist
Cedars-Sinai Health System
Los Angeles, California

Brenda R. Lance, RN, MSN
Nurse Coordinator
Ritzman Infusion Services
Akron, Ohio

Leonard L. Lance, RPh, BSPharm
Clinical Pharmacist
Lexi-Comp Inc
Hudson, Ohio

Jerrold B. Leikin, MD
Associate Director
Emergency Services
Rush Presbyterian-St Luke's Medical Center
Chicago, Illinois

Timothy F. Meiller, DDS, PhD
Professor
Department of Oral Medicine and Diagnostic Sciences
Baltimore College of Dental Surgery
Professor of Oncology
Greenebaum Cancer Center
University of Maryland at Baltimore
Baltimore, Maryland

Eugene S. Olsowka, MD, PhD
Pathologist
Institute of Pathology PC
Saginaw, Michigan

12

PREFACE

The *Clinician's Endodontic Handbook* was written because of the perceived need by the authors, that a quick reference guide to clinical endodontics was unavailable for the busy practitioner. Although there are several excellent textbooks on Endodontics, they often provide significantly more information, in much greater detail than what might be desired for the typical clinical situation. The authors have included numerous "Clinical Note" sections in most chapters to aid the practitioner while performing endodontics. The "Clinical Note" sections represent over 40 years of combined clinical experience between the authors. They are intended to help both the neophyte and the seasoned clinician, but primarily are included for the benefit of our patients. In addition, frequently asked questions have been included with the purpose of helping the practitioner communicate better with their patients and also for a better understanding of the practice of endodontics. The authors sincerely hope the *Clinician's Endodontic Handbook* will fill that void between theory and practical knowledge in the rapidly expanding field of endodontics.

Dr. Thom C. Dumsha
Dr. James L. Gutmann

ACKNOWLEDGMENTS

The *Clinician's Endodontic Handbook* exists in its present form as the result of the concerted efforts of the following individuals: Robert D. Kerscher, publisher and president of Lexi-Comp Inc; Lynn D. Coppinger, managing editor; Barbara F. Kerscher, production manager; David C. Marcus, director of information systems; Brad F. Bolinski, product manager; and Tracey J. Reinecke, graphic designer.

In addition, special acknowledgment is given to the Lexi-Comp staff for their contribution and/or participation in this handbook.

The authors wish to thank their families, friends, and colleagues who supported them in their efforts to complete this handbook.

Dr Dumsha would like, in particular, to thank his best friend and wife, Carol, for always being there. He would also like to recognize his mentors, Dr James Gutmann, who he considers "the clinician's academician and the academician's clinician"; and Dr Eric Hovland who he considers "the academician's academician." — TCD

"Thanks Marylou for your patience and understanding!" — JLG

SAFE WRITING

Health professionals and their support personnel frequently produce handwritten copies of information they see in print; therefore, such information is subjected to even greater possibilities for error or misinterpretation on the part of others. Thus, particular care must be given to how drug names and strengths are expressed when creating written healthcare documents.

The following are a few examples of safe writing rules suggested by the Institute for Safe Medication Practices, Inc.*

1. There should be a space between a number and its units as it is easier to read. There should be no periods after the abbreviations mg or mL.

Correct	Incorrect
10 mg	10mg
100 mg	100mg

2. Never place a decimal and a zero after a whole number (2 mg is correct and 2.0 mg is **incorrect**). If the decimal point is not seen because it falls on a line or because individuals are working from copies where the decimal point is not seen, this causes a tenfold overdose.

3. Just the opposite is true for numbers less than one. Always place a zero before a naked decimal (0.5 mL is correct, .5 mL is **incorrect**).

4. Never abbreviate the word unit. The handwritten U or u, looks like a 0 (zero), and may cause a tenfold overdose error to be made.

5. IU is not a safe abbreviation for international units. The handwritten IU looks like IV. Write out international units or use int. units.

6. Q.D. is not a safe abbreviation for once daily, as when the Q is followed by a sloppy dot, it looks like QID which means four times daily.

7. O.D. is not a safe abbreviation for once daily, as it is properly interpreted as meaning "right eye" and has caused liquid medications such as saturated solution of potassium iodide and Lugol's solution to be administered incorrectly. There is no safe abbreviation for once daily. It must be written out in full.

8. Do not use chemical names such as 6-mercaptopurine or 6-thioguanine, as sixfold overdoses have been given when these were not recognized as chemical names. The proper names of these drugs are mercaptopurine or thioguanine.

9. Do not abbreviate drug names (5FC, 6MP, 5-ASA, MTX, HCTZ, CPZ, PBZ, etc) as they are misinterpreted and cause error.

10. Do not use the apothecary system or symbols.

11. Do not abbreviate microgram as μg; instead use mcg as there is less likelihood of misinterpretation.

12. When writing an outpatient prescription, write a complete prescription. A complete prescription can prevent the prescriber, the pharmacist, and/or the patient from making a mistake and can eliminate the need for further clarification. The legible prescriptions should contain:

    a. patient's full name

    b. for pediatric or geriatric patients: their age (or weight where applicable)

    c. drug name, dosage form and strength; if a drug is new or rarely prescribed, print this information

    d. number or amount to be dispensed

    e. complete instructions for the patient, including the purpose of the medication

    f. when there are recognized contraindications for a prescribed drug, indicate to the pharmacist that you are aware of this fact (ie, when prescribing a potassium salt for a patient receiving an ACE inhibitor, write "K serum level being monitored")

*From "Safe Writing" by Davis NM, PharmD and Cohen MR, MS, Lecturers and Consultants for Safe Medication Practices, 1143 Wright Drive, Huntington Valley, PA 19006. Phone: (215) 947-7566.

Chapter I

Histology of Tooth and Supporting Periodontium

HISTOLOGY OF TOOTH AND SUPPORTING PERIODONTIUM

A. TEETH

- Constitute approximately 20% of the surface of the oral cavity
- Serve a number of functions, are commonly associated with mastication, speech, and aesthetics
- And supporting structures, made of a multitude of tissues, each having their own origin, purpose, and function
- Are attached to the bone by a fibrous ligament

B. ENAMEL

- Hard, acellular, inert tissue covers the anatomical tooth crown
- Formed by the ameloblast, a cell found only in the developing tooth bud
- Most highly mineralized tissue in the body consisting of 96% inorganic material – hydroxyapatite crystallites with traces of organic material enveloping each crystallite
- High inorganic content renders enamel vulnerable to demineralization in the acid environment of bacteria, leading to caries

---

* * * * * Clinical Note * * * * *

The smooth enamel surfaces can be reinforced against bacterial attack with fluoride applications. When the integrity of the enamel covering is compromised on the occlusal or biting surface of premolar or molar teeth, bonded sealants can be placed to prevent bacterial attack. Once the enamel is invaded or destroyed by bacteria or trauma, the body is unable to regenerate this tissue.

C. DENTIN

- Hard, elastic, yellowish white, avascular tissue immediately beneath the enamel that surrounds the dental pulp
- Connective organ responsible for dentin formation
- Formed by the odontoblast, a cell from the dental pulp (primitive dental papilla that governs tooth development)

- 70% mineralized with hydroxyapatite crystals, organic component is mainly fibrous protein collagen

- Tissue consists of closely packed tubules, 38-40,000 per square mm present in the coronal portion of the tooth, decreasing to 18-20,000 per square mm in the root portion

- Tubules contain fluid that may transport irritants and serve to transfer specific stimuli to the dental pulp

- Tubules may also undergo closure with aging or continuous challenges from bacteria or other oral entities (abrasion from tooth brushing, restorative procedures, or restorative materials)

D. PULP

- Soft, fibrous, connective tissue located in the central portion of the tooth in both the coronal chamber and root canals

- Has the following functions:

  - Forms the dentin

  - Supplies nutrition to the avascular dentin

  - Protects the tooth by giving the dentin its sensitivity

  - Repairs the dentin with new dentin when the pulp is challenged with insults

- Organizes from primitive dental papilla and undergoes organization during hard tissue formation (enamel and dentin)

- Highly vascular and innervated

- When irritated with bacterial products or bacteria themselves, or is subject to trauma or multiple dental procedures, removal (pulpectomy) and treatment (root canal treatment) is necessary to retain the tooth in the oral cavity

- Movement of bacterial products or bacteria from within the pulp to the supporting tissues (periradicular tissues) of the jaw cause inflammation and infection – commonly referred to as an abscess

---

***** Clinical Note *****

Diagnosis and treatment of an inflammatory/infectious process
in the dental pulp and supporting tissues of the jaw can
be found in Chapters III and XI, respectfully.

E. CEMENTUM

- Hard bone-like tissue, covers the external portion of the root, firmly cemented to the dentin

- Formed from the cementoblast, a cell that is recruited from the surrounding, supporting tissues

- Avascular and about 50% mineralized – hydroxyapatite and collagen

- Serves to anchor the tooth in the jawbone with bundles or groups of fibers running from the cementum to the bone and vice-versa

- Presence of cementum is essential to prevent the possibility of external root resorption (see Chapters XII and XIII)

- Regenerates from cells in the surrounding periodontal ligament and bone that serves as the source of cementoblast precursors

---

* * * * *   Clinical Note   * * * * *

When the cementum has been destroyed from periodontal disease, techniques of guided tissue regeneration (GTR) may be indicated to enhance or encourage cemental regeneration. Cementum is deposited routinely throughout life and will often alter the position of the apical foramen, which impacts on working length determination during root canal treatment. When the apical cementum has been removed during endodontic root-end surgery, regeneration can occur routinely once the etiology has been removed.

F. PERIODONTAL LIGAMENT

- Highly specialized connective tissue approximately 0.2-0.3 mm in width, situated between the tooth and jaw (alveolar) bone

- Principal functions: Connect the tooth to the jaw and support the tooth during the considerable forces of mastication

- Multiple groups of collagen fibers strategically placed at various angles between the tooth and the jawbone in order to adapt to the multitude of stresses placed on teeth during function

- Surrounds the root apex, can undergo rapid inflammation and degradation in the presence of bacteria or inflammatory products emanating from the dental pulp

***** Clinical Note *****

Evidence of the changes in the periodontal ligament from
inflammation and infection of pulpal origin can often be
observed or determined radiographically and clinically –
see Chapters III and IV. Radiographic changes and
clinical probings can determine the extent
of periodontal ligament loss when
periodontal disease is present.

G. ALVEOLAR BONE

- Makes up the alveolar (jaw) process that houses the teeth

- Consists of two types of bone: Spongy type (cancellous) and dense type (basal)

- Teeth are housed in spongy type of bone

- Spongy bone influenced rapidly by inflammation and infection, with destruction of the mineral content evident on the radiograph

***** Clinical Note *****

Bone will regenerate upon removal of the offending causes of
deterioration. This occurs routinely following nonsurgical
and surgical root canal treatment.

H. PERIODONTIUM

- Refers to a composite of periodontal ligament, cementum, and alveolar bone

***** Clinical Note *****

See Chapter XV on pulpal - periodontal interactions that
expand on the dynamic interplay between these
two tissues in the clinical setting.

FREQUENTLY ASKED QUESTIONS (FAQs)

1. *If the dental pulp can be the source of pain for the patient, why not just remove the pulp in all of the teeth and prevent toothaches?*

   The dental pulp provides important functions for the patient throughout life, such as the formation of reparative dentin, a sensory signal when irritants or bacteria may be invading the tooth, and proprioception during function.

2. *Following root canal treatment, can cementum be formed and seal the apical foramen of the root-treated tooth?*

   Yes — this is common following quality root canal treatment, especially when the root filling material is not protruding beyond the cleaned and shaped pulpal space. The chance for complete regeneration with cementum is negated when the root canal system has not been cleaned, shaped, and/or obturated thoroughly within the confines of the canal system.

Chapter II

Common Access, Root, Chamber, and Canal Configurations

COMMON ACCESS, ROOT, CHAMBER, AND CANAL CONFIGURATIONS

A. MAXILLARY ARCH

Maxillary Central Incisors

- Single root

- Usually straight root

- Probability of 1 canal ~100%

- Typical length ~23-25 mm

- When curvature of root occurs, usually toward distal

- Usually erupts around age 7-8

- Chamber is triangular in design with high pulp horns on mesial and distal aspects of chamber

- Lingual ledge or lingual bulge often present

---

* * * * *   Clinical Note   * * * * *

Lingual ledge is important since failure to remove it during access preparation may result, during instrumentation, in a migration of files toward the labial.

- Access opening is triangular in shape

---

* * * * *   Clinical Note   * * * * *

Discoloration of incisor teeth, after root canal therapy, is not uncommon; however, it is almost completely preventable. Failure to remove entirely the mesial and distal pulp horns during access preparation will cause this tissue to eventually break down. The products of this tissue then diffuse into the dentinal tubules and cause a brown-gray discoloration of the dentin.

Maxillary Lateral Incisors

- Single root
- Often the apical one-third to one-quarter of the root curves or dilacerates
- Probability of 1 canal ~100%
- Typical length ~22-23 mm
- Curvature usually occurs toward the distal
- Usually erupts around age 7-9
- Chamber is similar to central incisors but proportionately smaller
- Lingual ledge may also be present, but is usually not clinically significant
- Access opening is triangular, similar to maxillary central incisors, and proportionately smaller in the middle third of the lingual surface of the tooth

Maxillary Canine

- Single root
- Straight root; however, often the apical one-third to one-quarter of the root curves or dilacerates
- Probability of 1 canal ~100%
- Typical length ~24-27 mm

---

* * * * *   Clinical Note   * * * * *

Canine teeth, because of the anatomy of the canal system (oval/elliptical), their extreme length, and the size of the canal system, are probably the most difficult anterior tooth in which to perform root canal therapy. Open access sufficiently in size and for straight-line-access to accommodate the larger diameter files.

- Curvature or dilacerations usually to lingual, labial, or distal
- Usually erupts around age 11
- Chamber is usually elliptical or oval in shape
- Lingual ledge may be present, usually not clinically significant
- Access opening oval in shape, on the lingual surface, and should be in the middle third of the tooth both mesiodistally and incisal-apically

Maxillary First Premolar

- Single or 2-rooted system
- Root fusion can range from coronal half of root to complete fusion of entire root length
- Usually 2 canals (buccal and palatal) >85% of the time
- When 2 roots, usually separate foramen
- Buccal root usually curved more than palatal root
- Palatal root usually larger of the 2 roots
- Typical length ~21-22 mm
- Usually erupts around age 10-11
- Chamber usually oval in shape
- There are often ledges of calcification on the buccal and/or lingual walls just coronal to the orifice that may inhibit straight-line-access to the canal system

---

* * * * *   Clinical Note   * * * * *

The pulp chamber in maxillary premolars, particularly in the first premolar is often "skewed" to the mesial or distal with respect to the anatomical crown. Awareness of this fact will prevent an access opening preparation that destroys more tooth structure than is actually required to gain proper visibility of both canals and straight-line-access.

- Chamber usually oval in shape
- Access opening oval in shape on the occlusal surface and should be in the middle third of the tooth both mesiodistally and buccolingually
- Buccal and lingual cusps should not be undermined during access opening preparation

Maxillary Second Premolar

- Single or 2-rooted system but usually single
- Root fusion can range from coronal half of root to complete fusion of entire root length
- Highest probability — 1 root and 1 canal
- Occasionally will have 2 or, very rarely, 3 canals
- When 2 canals are present, usually 2 foramen
- Typical length ~21-22 mm
- Usually erupts around age 10-12

***** **Clinical Note** *****

The apical 1/3 to 1/4 of many maxillary premolars (both 1st and 2nd) roots will dilacerate. Examine the radiographs of these teeth very closely before cleaning and shaping and proceed with great caution if a dilaceration is present. Maintaining a smaller master apical file size will prevent numerous cleaning and shaping errors in these teeth.

- Chamber usually oval in shape

- Access opening is oval on the occlusal surface and should be in the middle third of the tooth both mesiodistally and buccolingually

- The buccal and lingual cusps should not be undermined during access opening preparation

***** **Clinical Note** *****

Ideal access openings in maxillary premolar teeth should allow an explorer to penetrate down the buccal and/or lingual surface of the access opening directly into the orifice of the canal.

Maxillary First Molar

- Usually a 3-root system, can rarely have 4 distinct roots

- Mesiobuccal (MB) root, distobuccal (DB) root, and palatal (P) root

   - MB root often curves toward distal in apical 1/3

   - DB root usually straight but can have distal or buccal curvature in apical 1/3

   - P root is the largest and often has a buccal curvature in the apical 1/3

***** **Clinical Note** *****

Before instrumenting the palatal root of a maxillary first molar, examine the apical 1/3 of the working length file of this root to determine if there is a curvature in the apical 1/3. This curvature, if in a buccal direction, cannot be determined by radiographic evidence. Failure to note this will result in an inaccurately short working length and a high potential for perforation of the canal system.

- Palatal root will occasionally have 2 canals present, but high probability of one
- Distobuccal root will have only 1 canal system
- Mesiobuccal root will have very high probability of 2 canals – mesiobuccal and mesiopalatal (MP)

---

* * * * *   Clinical Note   * * * * *

Because of the extremely high probability of a second MB canal, it should always be assumed that it is present. It can be located within 1-2 mm of the mesiobuccal canal or at a midpoint between the palatal orifice and the mesiobuccal orifice.

- Mesiopalatal canal will be found palatal to the mesiobuccal canal orifice
- Mesiopalatal will usually exit into the mesiobuccal canal or become severely calcified as to prevent its complete negotiation
- Mesiopalatal is usually a very small and torturous canal system

---

* * * * *   Clinical Note   * * * * *

Exercise caution when cleaning and shaping the mesiopalatal canal system because of its size, calcification, and curvature. The master apical file size of the canal system generally need not be larger than a 25 K file.

- Typical length of MB and DB roots ~19-22 mm
- Typical length of palatal root ~22-25 mm
- Usually erupts around age 6-7
- Chamber is usually triangular to square in shape

---

* * * * *   Clinical Note   * * * * *

In elderly patients or in teeth with an extensive history of restorative procedures, the pulp chamber can become extremely calcified. In many cases, the only method for determining that the pulp chamber has been properly accessed is by noting a discoloration on the floor of the chamber.

***** **Clinical Note** *****

In cases where the radiographic presentation of a pulp
chamber is severely calcified, the distance from occlusal
surface to pulp chamber should be measured on the
radiograph with a periodontal probe. By knowing this
measurement, the access opening depth can then be
maintained only to this distance and the probability
of a furcation perforation becomes highly unlikely.

- Access opening is triangular to slightly square on the occlusal
  surface
- Access preparation should be distal to the mesial marginal
  ridge, within the middle third buccolingually, and mesial to the
  transverse ridge

    - The transverse ridge should not be undermined during
      access opening preparation

    - The access opening need not extend too far mesially as to
      undermine the mesial marginal ridge

***** **Clinical Note** *****

All too commonly, it is assumed incorrectly that the
mesiobuccal canal orifice is more mesial than its actual
location. The identification of the MB canal should be
the last aspect of access preparation so as to avoid
inadvertent destruction of mesial tooth structure.
If palatal and distobuccal canal orifices are first
identified, the mesiobuccal canal will be more
easily discovered without the unnecessary
removal of essential tooth structure.

***** **Clinical Note** *****

There are often ledges of calcifications or cervical ledges on
the buccal and/or lingual wall just coronal to the orifice
of the canals that may inhibit straight-line-access
to the canal system if not removed during
access preparation.

Maxillary Second Molar

- Usually a 3-root system
- Mesiobuccal root, distobuccal root, and palatal root
  - MB root often curves toward distal in apical 1/3
  - DB root usually straight, but can have mesial or distal curvature in apical 1/3
  - P root is the largest and may have a buccal curvature in the apical 1/3
- Palatal root will have 1 canal system
- Distobuccal root will have only 1 canal system
- Root structure is often more fused than the maxillary first molar
- Mesiobuccal root of the second molar will have lower probability of 2 canals than the MB root of the maxillary first molar

---

* * * * * Clinical Note * * * * *

Because of the potential (although lower than the maxillary first molar) of a MP canal, always assume that it is present and verify or negate its presence. It will usually be located between the mesiobuccal canal orifice and the palatal canal orifice.

  - MP will be found palatal to the mesiobuccal canal orifice
  - MP will exit into the mesiobuccal canal or become severely calcified as to prevent its complete negotiation
  - MP is usually a very small and torturous canal system
- Typical length of MB and DB roots ~19-22 mm
- Typical length of palatal root ~21-23 mm
- Usually erupts around age 12-13
- Chamber is usually less triangular and more oval in shape than the maxillary first molar
- Access opening is triangular but becomes more straightened in a mesiobuccal-palatal direction
- Access preparation should be distal to the mesial marginal ridge, within the middle third buccolingually, and mesial to the transverse ridge
  - The transverse ridge should not be undermined during access opening preparation
  - The access opening begins slightly more distal than in the first molar because of the location of the canal and root structure

Maxillary Third Molar

- Usually a 3-root system, but anatomy is typically very unusual; not uncommon to have only 1 or 2 roots

- Mesiobuccal root, distobuccal root, and palatal root when 3 roots are present

  - MB root often curves toward distal in apical 1/3

  - DB root usually has a mesial or distal curvature in apical 1/3

  - Palatal root is the largest and may have a buccal curvature in the apical 1/3

- Palatal root will have 1 canal system

- Mesiobuccal and distobuccal root will have only 1 canal system

- Root structure is often fused

- Mesiobuccal root of the third molar will have extremely low probability of 2 canals

- Typical length of MB and DB roots ~18-22 mm

- Typical length of palatal root ~18-23 mm

- Usually erupts around age 18-21

- Chamber is usually less triangular and more oval in shape than the maxillary second molar

- Access opening is somewhat triangular, but is more often rotated as the DB canal orifice becomes more aligned with the palatal canal

- Access preparation can begin in the central fossae and proceed in a buccopalatal direction

---

* * * * *   Clinical Note   * * * * *

In maxillary second and third molars, the orifices of the palatal
canal and, in particular, the MB and DB canals, are in close
approximation to each other on the floor of the pulp chamber.
Often, the 2 buccal canals will have one common
orifice that will separate into 2 separate canals.
No instrumentation is performed until both canals
are identified. Instrumentation of either canal
without the knowledge of the other canal
will often result in permanent blockage
of the untreated canal.

B. MANDIBULAR ARCH

Mandibular Central and Lateral Incisors

- Mandibular central and lateral incisors are nearly identical in their morphology
- Usually straight roots, although they may have slight dilacerations in the apical 1/3
- Relatively high probability of 2 canals
  - Labial (facial) canal and lingual canal
  - May have a common orifice near CEJ
  - When 2 canals are present, there is a very high probability that both lingual and facial canals join and exit with a common foramen

---

***** **Clinical Note** *****

There is a high probability of 2 canals in mandibular incisor teeth. If 2 are present, the canal most overlooked is the lingual. Often, the access opening must be extended more lingually in order to obtain straight-line-access to the lingual orifice and the canal system. In addition, all working length films taken of mandibular incisors should be exposed at a slight mesial or distal angle to confirm the presence or absence of a second canal.

- Typical length ~21-22 mm
- When curvature of the roots occur, the apical 1/3 usually bends slightly toward the lingual
- Usually erupt around age 6-8
- Chamber is triangular to oval in design with high pulp horns on mesial and distal aspects of chamber in younger patients
- Lingual ledge or lingual bulge may be present which restricts visualization of the canal orifice and prevents straight-line-access of the canal system

Mandibular Canine

- Usually a single root
- Straight root morphology; however, when curvature occurs, the apical 1/3 often curves toward the distal
- Very high probability of 1 canal; however, 2 canals are not rare

---

* * * * *   Clinical Note   * * * * *

If a patient has an unusually large number of roots and/or
canals in one particular tooth group (mandibular premolars), there is a higher probability that they will
have other teeth with multiple roots and/or
canals (mandibular canines,
mandibular incisors).

- Typical length ~25-26 mm

---

* * * * *   Clinical Note   * * * * *

Because of the morphology and arch position of mandibular
canine teeth, there are potential problems during access of
this tooth group. In addition, because of their extreme length,
and the size of the canal system they can provide great
difficulty during instrumentation. As with the maxillary
canine teeth, the access must be opened sufficiently
in size for straight-line-access in order to accommodate the larger diameter files that will be
required to properly clean and shape
the canal system.

- Usually erupts around age 9-10
- Chamber is usually elliptical or oval in shape
- Lingual ledge may be present
- Access opening is oval in shape on the lingual surface and
  should be in the middle third of the tooth both mesiodistally
  and incisal-apically

Mandibular First Premolar

- Usually a single root
- Usually 1 canal, 2 canals are not uncommon, although 3
  canals are rare
- If 2 canals are present, relatively high probability that they will
  exit with separate foramen
- Typical length ~21-22 mm
- Usually erupts around age 10-12
- Chamber is usually oval to rounded in shape

***** **Clinical Note** *****

The pulp chamber in mandibular premolars is often quite small. In addition, mandibular premolars have an anatomical crown and occlusal surface that is canted toward the lingual. These two factors in the presence of a rubber dam can prevent visualization of the long axis of the tooth. It is within the scope of endodontic practice to perform an access opening in these teeth or in others without the rubber dam in place. After the access opening is completed, the rubber dam should then be placed over the tooth before any files or other instruments are introduced into the mouth.

- Access opening is oval to rounded in shape on the occlusal surface and should be in the middle third of the tooth both mesiodistally and buccolingually
- The buccal cusp should not be destroyed or undermined during access opening preparation

Mandibular Second Premolar

- Single rooted system
- Higher probability of only 1 canal than mandibular first premolar, but not rare to have 2 canals present (<15%)
- Three canals are very rare
- When 2 canals are present, usually 2 foramen
- Typical length ~21-22 mm
- Usually erupts around age 11-12

***** **Clinical Note** *****

The apical 1/3 to 1/4 of many mandibular premolar (both 1st and 2nd) roots will dilacerate. Examine the radiographs of these teeth very closely before beginning instrumentation and proceed with great caution if a dilaceration is present. Maintaining a smaller master apical file size will prevent numerous cleaning and shaping errors in these teeth.

- Chamber is usually oval in shape
- Access opening is oval on the occlusal surface and should be in the middle third of the tooth both mesiodistally and buccolingually
- The buccal and lingual cusps should not be undermined during access opening preparation

```
* * * * *   Clinical Note   * * * * *

Ideal access openings in mandibular premolar teeth should
allow an explorer to slide down the buccal and/or lingual
surface of the access opening and to penetrate with
the explorer tip directly into the orifice of the canal.
```

Mandibular First Molar

- Usually a 2-root system, can rarely have 3 distinct roots (usually found in Asian population with a distinct buccal or distobuccal root)
- Mesial root and distal root
    - Mesial root often curves toward distal in apical 1/3
    - Distal root may be straight, or curve in a mesial direction, occasionally will curve distally
- Mesial root will routinely have 2 canals
    - Mesial canals usually exit with separate foramen
- Distal root will have only 1 canal but high probability of 2 separate canals (distobuccal and distolingual)

```
* * * * *   Clinical Note   * * * * *

Because of the extremely high probability of a second distal
canal, assume that it is present until proven otherwise. The
access opening should be more square than the classical
triangular shape if there are 2 distal canals.
```

```
* * * * *   Clinical Note   * * * * *

Exercise caution when instrumenting the mesial root canal
system because of its size, potential calcification, and
curvature. The master apical file size of the canal
system after instrumentation generally need
not be larger than a 25 K file.
```

- Typical length of mesial root ~21 mm
- Typical length of distal root ~22-23 mm
- Usually erupts around age 6-7
- Chamber is usually triangular to square in shape
- Access opening is triangular to slightly square on the occlusal surface

- Access preparation should be distal to the mesial marginal ridge and primarily within the mesial half of the occlusal surface; although the distal extension of the access opening should extend into the distal half of the tooth

---

***** Clinical Note *****

Do not assume that the mesial canals are more mesial than their actual location. The identification of the mesial canals should occur after the pulp chamber has been identified by access first into the center of the chamber. The tooth structure should be removed cautiously toward the mesial aspect of the tooth to identify the 2 mesial canals. Since the distal canal is the largest, it is usually most easily identified.

Mandibular Second Molar

- Usually a 2-root system
- Mesial root and distal root
    - Mesial root often curves toward distal in apical 1/3
    - Distal root usually has a distal curvature associated with it
- Distal root usually will have only 1 canal system
- Root structure is often more fused than the mandibular first molar
- Mesial root of the second molar will have lower probability of 2 canals than the mesial root of the mandibular first molar

---

***** Clinical Note *****

Because of the potential (although lower than the mandibular first molar) of a second mesial canal, assume that it is present and verify or negate its presence. It is not uncommon for the mesial root of the second molar to have one orifice centered between the buccal and lingual walls of the pulp chamber. This one orifice will lead into 2 separate canal systems.

- Mesial canals are very small and often calcified
    - In most cases, master apical file size should be no larger than a 25-30 K file
- Typical length of mesial and distal roots ~20-21 mm
- Usually erupts around age 11-13
- Chamber is usually triangular in shape

- Access opening is triangular, but becomes more straightened in a mesiodistal direction if 2 separate orifices are not present in the mesial root

- Access preparation should be distal to the mesial marginal ridge and primarily within the mesial half of the occlusal surface, although the distal extension of the access opening should extend into the distal half of the tooth

---

* * * * *   Clinical Note   * * * * *

Both the mandibular first and second molars may have a "C-shaped" canal system. This type of anatomy of the canal systems can result in a blending of the mesial and distal canals. The result is a very wide canal orifice of both mesial and distal canals. Proper cleaning and shaping of this canal system is dependent upon not only proper instrumentation, but to a high degree, proper irrigant to dissolve tissue that files may not be able to remove. Care should be exercised during cleaning and shaping of these "C-shaped" canal systems to remove the tissue as completely as possible.

Mandibular Third Molar

- Usually a 2-root system but anatomy is typically very unusual, not uncommon to have only 1 root

- Mesial root and distal root when 2 roots are present

  - Mesial root and distal root often curve toward distal in apical 1/2

- Mesial and distal root usually will have only 1 canal system in each root

- Root structure is often fused

- Mesial root of the third molar will have extremely low probability of 2 canals

- Typical length of mesial and distal roots ~18-22 mm

- Usually erupts around age 18-21

- Chamber is usually less triangular and more oval in shape than the mandibular second molar

- Access opening is triangular to oval in shape

- Pulp chamber tends to be very large and very deep

FREQUENTLY ASKED QUESTIONS (FAQs)

1. ***Which teeth commonly have more than 1 canal?***

    Always rule out multiple canals in both mandibular premolars, maxillary second premolars, distal canals of mandibular first molar, and the mesiopalatal root of the maxillary first molar.

2. ***If the tooth is malpositioned, can the access opening be made from a different tooth surface?***

    Yes, to facilitate straight-line access to the pulp chamber. For example, the access opening can be made on the facial or incisal surface of a rotated anterior tooth. Incorrect access openings or improper placement will lead to improper ability to find and C&S the root canals and a high potential for ledging and other iatrogenic errors.

Chapter III

Diagnosis of Pulp and Periradicular Diseases

DIAGNOSIS OF PULP AND PERIRADICULAR DISEASES

A. DIAGNOSIS

6-Step Process

> ***** Clinical Note *****
>
> Determine reversible or irreversible symptoms – then diagnose vital or nonvital conditions of pulp

- Chief complaint
- Medical history
- Information gathering about symptoms
- Reproduce symptoms, if possible – additional tests / visual examination
- Make diagnosis
- Verify diagnosis with treatment

Chief Complaint

- Listen to patient's own words about symptoms and <u>document</u> exactly what patient stated regarding their pain

> ***** Clinical Note *****
>
> After listening to the patient's chief complaint (eg, if patient complains about "cold sensitivity"), **first step** in making the most probable diagnosis is reproducing the patient's chief complain. In this example, reproduce the painful sensation to cold.

Medical History

- Take a thorough medical history before any clinical tests / examination / radiographs, or dental staff and/or clinician performs additional procedures

Subjective Information Gathering

- Stimulus of pain
    - cold-heat-chewing
- Frequency of pain
    - several times/hour/day/continuous
- Duration of pain
    - minutes/hours
- Severity of pain
    - is patient taking analgesics?
    - are analgesics beneficial?
    - what type of analgesics relieve the pain?
- Spontaneity of pain
    - extremely important with respect to determining accurate diagnosis

---

***** Clinical Note *****

Spontaneous pain indicates high probability of an irreversible condition – not necessarily irreversible pulpitis, but an irreversible condition (patient in need of endodontics or other definitive dental services).

Reproduce Symptoms – Cold Tests / Heat Tests / Percussion

- All cold tests are **not** equal
- Currently available
    - Ice (frozen water)
    - Ethyl chloride (dichlorodifloromethane)
    - FRIGI-DENT (Ellman)
    - Endo Ice (Hygienic Corp)
    - CO_2 Ice/Snow (Myco-Union Broach)

***** Clinical Note *****

Do not routinely use ice or ethyl chloride as cold tests – these do not achieve adequately low temperatures.

- Ideal heat test response is obtained by *individual isolation* of each tooth to be tested with rubber dam

- – Use a 3-5 mL endodontic irrigating syringe filled with hot water/coffee/etc, and flow hot liquid over each isolated tooth

- – Remember to proceed slowly (waiting 45-120 seconds between testing) to assure an accurate response

- Burlew disk on slow speed will also produce heat

  - – Place disk on metal restoration (if possible) vs tooth structure to obtain better response

- Heat stick compound is also another method for thermal testing of teeth

  - – Ensure teeth are wetted before placing compound to prevent sticking of the compound and unnecessary pain for the patient

B. CLASSIFICATION OF CLINICAL PULPAL STATES

Normal Pulp

COMMON CLINICAL PRESENTATIONS

- Little or no sensitivity to cold/heat

- Cold/heat response lasts ~3-10 seconds

- Tooth may be percussion-sensitive due to high occlusion

Reversible Pulpitis

COMMON CLINICAL PRESENTATIONS

- Often a first-time complaint by a patient

- History of recent restoration (usually an amalgam, composite, crown preparation within several days to a couple of weeks)

- Patient reports sensitivity to air, cold liquids/foods, less frequently hot foods/liquids

- Symptoms resolve quickly after stimulus is removed

- No radiographic changes

```
* * * * *   Clinical Note   * * * * *
```

Patients commonly state a chief complaint of sensitivity to
both hot and cold liquids/foods; however, *vast majority
of time patients have sensitivity to* **cold** *and not to
hot* (during late stages of IP, patients are
typically heat-sensitive).

Irreversible Pulpitis (IP)

COMMON CLINICAL PRESENTATIONS

- EPT/cold elicit positive response

```
* * * * *   Clinical Note   * * * * *
```

Remember, the absolute value of the numbers on EPT devices are
meaningless. The only exception to this rule: if a response is
obtained from EPT test that is close to the upper limit
of the testing device (eg, 72-79 on the Analytic
Technology EPT), retest the tooth as this is
likely a false-positive response resulting
from too wet a field on the tooth.

- History of spontaneous pain
- Classical symptoms of <u>lingering and severe pain</u> upon removal
  of cold/heat stimulus
- Chief complaint of pain to cold liquids/foods which lasts several
  minutes or longer
- In late stages of IP, hot liquids/foods become the chief
  complaint and are the primary source of pain

```
* * * * *   Clinical Note   * * * * *
```

When performing cold/heat tests on potential irreversibly inflamed
teeth, <u>always wait at least 45-120 seconds</u> between testing
suspected teeth. Often, the severely painful throbbing
response that occurs after the immediate response
to the cold/heat stimulus is not produced
immediately. <u>Rapid testing of multiple
teeth will result in confusion with
respect to the correct
etiology.</u>

- Patient often believes they can identify which tooth is etiology

- Pain often increases in duration and/or frequency over days to weeks

- Pain is often diffuse and radiates to adjacent anatomical areas

    - Patients may complain of pain in TMJ area/preauricular area

- Pain can be masked and referred pain will appear to be in opposite arch from etiology

    - Referred pain will rarely, if ever, cross midline

- Tooth may be percussion-sensitive but often in early stages of IP is not

- Patients are often taking analgesics, as pain levels are usually moderate to severe

- Radiographic presentation of periradicular area may be WNL or have a slightly widened periodontal ligament space around one or more roots

    - Occasional erosion of lamina dura

Necrotic Pulp

COMMON CLINICAL PRESENTATIONS

- Symptoms often are similar to IP

    - Spontaneous pain

    - Occasionally severe pain to hot liquids/foods (late stages of IP/early necrotic pulp)

    - Radiating pain to TMJ

    - Diffuse throughout arch

- Spontaneous pain or complete absence of pain

- Patient may present with draining sinus tract in which case the patient will usually be asymptomatic and will likely remain asymptomatic
- Percussion sensitivity may or may not be present
- Radiographic presentation may be similar to IP
  - Little or no radiographic changes
  - May have definitive radiographic changes such as frank widened PDL and loss of lamina dura
- Radiographic changes may be obvious
  - Small to large radiolucent lesion around apex of one or more roots, depending on tooth group

---

* * * * *   **Clinical Note**   * * * * *

A significant amount of the mandibular cortical plate must be lost on either the buccal or lingual side before radiographic evidence of a lesion will appear.

---

* * * * *   **Clinical Note**   * * * * *

Patient may have experienced a previous episode of pain (mild/moderate to severe) but also may be asymptomatic with IP and/or necrotic pulpal states.

C. CLASSIFICATION OF PERIRADICULAR STATES

Acute Periradicular Periodontitis

- Inflammation of the tissues surrounding the root of pulpal origin
- Patient cannot bite on tooth and/or painful to percussion
- May or may not exhibit radiographic changes in radicular tissues

Chronic Periradicular Periodontitis

- Presence of a radiolucency
- Patient is asymptomatic

Chronic Suppurative Periradicular Periodontitis

- Presence of a radiolucency and a sinus tract
- Patient is usually asymptomatic

D. CLASSIFICATION OF PERIRADICULAR LESIONS

- Extremely high probability that vast majority (90%) of periradicular lesions are granulomas, cysts, or abscesses

---

***** **Clinical Note** *****

The histological nature of most periradicular lesions (cyst, granulomas, etc) **cannot** be diagnosed from a radiograph, regardless of their appearance.

***** **Clinical Note** *****

A classification of periradicular lesions based on radiographic appearance and/or patient symptoms/signs is without merit and treatment should not be premised on arbitrary names provided for periradicular states, but rather the clinical condition of the patient.

- Additional radiolucent lesions (see Chapter IV on Radiographic Interpretation)

  - Ameloblastic fibroma

  - Ameloblastoma

  - Central giant cell granuloma

  - Dentigerous cyst

  - Globulomaxillary cyst

  - Keratocyst

  - Lateral periodontal cyst

  - Median palatal cyst

  - Nasopalatine duct cyst

  - Primordial cyst

  - Residual cyst

  - Scar tissue

  - Traumatic bone cyst

- Additional radiopaque lesions
    - Cementoma (PCD)
    - Condensing osteitis (CO)
    - Fibrous dysplasia
    - Odontoma
    - Ossifying fibroma
    - Osteoblastoma
    - Osteosarcoma

E. MICROBIOLOGY OF PULPAL AND PERIRADICULAR DISEASES

- No specific bacteria have been absolutely associated with specific endodontic symptoms
- Common bacteria are *Lactobacilli, Streptococcus*, and *Actinomyces*
- Common root canal and periradicular bacteria are *Porphyromonas, Lactobacillus, Fusobacterium, Peptostreptococcus, Actinomycosis, Prevotella*, and *Bacteroides*
- Black pigmented bacteria are thought to have one of the highest associations with symptomatic teeth

FREQUENTLY ASKED QUESTIONS (FAQs)

1. *What is an irreversible pulpitis?*

    This condition occurs when the pulp becomes significantly inflamed from a variety of reasons. The causative agents can be decay in the tooth, trauma from a blow, fracture of tooth structure, or simple restorative procedures such as amalgam, composite, or tooth preparation for a crown. Whenever decay is removed or the tooth is prepared for a "filling" (composite or amalgam restorations), a "cap" (crown and/or bridgework), or other procedures that may affect the "nerve" (pulp), the potential for pulpal inflammation is high. Depending upon the initial state of the pulp (normal, reversible pulpitis, or irreversible pulpitis), additional insult will result in pain and inflammation of the "nerve" of the tooth.

    If the inflammation to too severe, then an irreversible pulpitis will result, analogous to one more straw that breaks the camel's back. If the pulp becomes irreversibly inflamed, symptoms will develop and the patient will be in moderate to severe pain.

2. *What is a necrotic pulp?*

When the "tooth nerve", which is actually the nerve, blood vessels, and all of the cellular and noncellular contents within the pulp, becomes severely damaged and dies, the pulp is considered to be necrotic. This is similar to when your skin dies and scabs over and sloughs off from the underlying layer when you scrape your arm. Only in the tooth, there is nowhere for this tissue to go and therefore it has to stay inside the tooth. Also, the soft tissue within the tooth does not have as much help to fix the "nerve" as does your skin or other tissues on your body. The tissues "break down" and can sometimes form an abscess because of the bacteria that live inside the tooth. These bacteria are part of the reason that a tooth hurts when it becomes necrotic or when the tissue dies. These bacteria can become very serious threats to your overall health and must be removed as soon as possible.

3. *What does it mean when a tooth hurts to biting?*

If no recent restorative work has been performed on the tooth or a history of trauma or parafunctional habits, then the likelihood of pulpal inflammation extending into the periradicular tissues is high. Another possibility is that the tooth may be fractured.

4. *I had a toothache in the past but my tooth doesn't hurt anymore, why do I need a root canal?*

During the time that you had pain, the pulp was undergoing inflammation that ultimately was irreversible in nature and may have caused the death or necrosis of the pulp. A thorough examination of the pulp and periradicular tissues will help to clarify the most probable state of these tissues. It no longer hurts because following an inflammatory challenge, the pulp may have died or become chronically inflamed exhibiting little or no symptoms.

Chapter IV

Radiographic Interpretation of Alterations in Normal Tooth Structure and Surrounding Bone

RADIOGRAPHIC INTERPRETATION OF ALTERATIONS IN NORMAL TOOTH STRUCTURE AND SURROUNDING BONE

A. ALTERATION IN THE CORONAL TOOTH STRUCTURE

- Radiolucent areas under amalgam, composite, or other restorations indicate a high probability of recurrent decay

- Irreversible pulpitis does not necessarily correlate with radiolucent areas within the coronal aspect of the tooth

---

* * * * *   Clinical Note   * * * * *

Often an irreversibly inflamed pulp is due to multiple insults to the tooth over a long period of time. In these cases, the radiographic picture of both the coronal and periradicular area will be within normal limits, thereby requiring a diagnosis based solely on patient symptoms and clinical signs.

- Depending upon the angle of exposure (especially in maxillary teeth), the pulp chamber may appear to be completely calcified, although clinically it may be a normal size or only slightly reduced from normal

- In single-rooted canal systems, the coronal third of the root may appear to become calcified and is called a "fast break" which indicates one of three events

  1. A large pulp chamber has split into two canals

  2. One large canal has split into two canals

  3. Two separate canals that were superimposed on each other have split into different directions

  - These are most often seen in mandibular 1st and 2nd premolar teeth

- Radiolucent areas on one or both sides of the CEJ area are often misinterpreted for decay when in all probability this area is a radiographic artifact known as "cervical burnout"

- Other than that associated with carious lesions, a necrotic pulp will not demonstrate any coronal radiographic changes that can aid in developing a diagnosis

B. PATHOSIS OF PULPAL ORIGIN AROUND THE ROOT

Irreversible Pulpitis

- Radiographic periradicular changes are often not present in early stages of irreversible pulpitis

- Patients may have a long-standing history of pain (several weeks to several months) without frank changes in the periradicular bony structure

- Often, the first radiographic signs of an IP are a slightly widened periodontal ligament width and/or a thickened lamina dura

- The lamina dura is often lost in small areas where the periodontal ligament has become widened

---

* * * * *   Clinical Note   * * * * *

The inability to detect a complete lamina dura around a root
does not indicate that there is pathosis present. If one
examines most periradicular radiographs, it is unlikely that a
complete lamina dura can be detected for the entire root.
This occurs because of the angulation of the roots
and the inability of one radiograph to capture
the entire angle of a root, such that the
complete lamina dura can
be detected.

Necrotic Pulp

- Periradicular changes with a necrotic pulp may range from no changes in the bony architecture, to mild radiolucent changes, to a frank radiolucent lesion

- It is not uncommon for a necrotic pulp in a multirooted tooth to demonstrate only one root as having a radiolucency or periradicular changes from normal

- Changes in the periradicular area will occur more rapidly in maxillary teeth than in mandibular teeth

  - The density of the cortical bone that must be destroyed in maxillary teeth is usually significantly less than in mandibular teeth

- Less than 13% of the cortical plate must be destroyed before a lesion will appear radiolucent

```
* * * * *    Clinical Note    * * * * *

When a sinus tract is present, there is a perforation of the
cortical bone; however, the area may be quite small
in diameter and will not necessarily be
detectable radiographically.
```

C. RADIOLUCENT AND RADIOPAQUE LESIONS

Radiolucent	Radiopaque (Some are RL at onset)
Ameloblastoma	Cementoma (PCD)
Ameloblastic Fibroma	Condensing Osteitis (CO)
Central Giant Cell Granuloma	Fibrous Dysplasia
Dentigerous Cyst	Odontoma
Globulomaxillary Cyst	Ossifying Fibroma
Keratocyst	Osteoblastoma
Lateral Periodontal Cyst	Osteosarcoma
Median Palatal Cyst	
Nasopalatine Duct Cyst	
Primordial Cyst	
Residual Cyst	
Scar Tissue	
Traumatic Bone Cyst	

D. RADIOLUCENT LESIONS

Ameloblastoma

- Occurs in both the maxilla and mandible; however, propensity for posterior mandible

- Can be unilocular or multilocular

- Aggressive lesion but benign

- Occurs more frequently in middle adulthood

- Patients are symptom-free

- May cause severe expansion of bone and destruction of both tooth structure and bone

- Teeth usually respond normally to pulp testing

Ameloblastic Fibroma

- Occurs in younger patients
- Primarily in the mandible posterior region
- Can be unilocular or multilocular, but usually multilocular
- Teeth usually respond normally to pulp testing
- Usually a very slow growing lesion
- Patients are usually asymptomatic

Central Giant Cell Granuloma

- Usually occurs in the region around the mandibular premolars and anterior teeth
- Occurs in young patients to young adults
- May be an aggressive type of lesion
- Can be unilocular or multilocular
- Causes destruction of the bone and/or expansion of the mandible
- May cause resorption of the dentition and/or tooth movement

Dentigerous Cyst

- Usually occurs in the region of unerupted or impacted third molars and maxillary canines
- Occurs in young patients to young adults
- Usually unilocular
- Can be very destructive to surrounding bone
- Can cause resorption of radicular tooth structure
- Patients are usually asymptomatic unless lesion becomes excessively large and begins to displace teeth or cause swelling of soft tissue
- Teeth usually respond normally to pulp testing

Globulomaxillary Cyst

- Considered a "fissural cyst"
- Occurs between the maxillary canine and lateral incisor
- Usually unilocular
- Some suggest the cyst may cause divergence of radicular tooth structure of canine and incisor

- Patients are asymptomatic
- Does not cause destruction of radicular tooth structure
- Teeth respond normally to pulp testing

Keratocyst (Odontogenic Keratocyst)

- Occurs primarily in the mandibular posterior region
- Found at any age
- May be unilocular or multilocular
- High tendency to reoccur
- Patients may become symptomatic as swelling increases and causes pressure
- Teeth usually respond normally to pulp testing
- May have both bone and tooth resorption
- May be associated with basal cell nevus syndrome

Lateral Periodontal Cyst

- Occurs primarily in the mandibular canine and premolar areas
- May be unilocular (most often) or multilocular
- Usually no resorption of tooth structure
- Teeth respond normally to pulp testing
- Patients are usually asymptomatic

Median Palatal Cyst

- Controversial as to its true existence
- Occurs in the midline region of the maxilla posterior to the anterior teeth
- Usually unilocular
- Seen more often in adult patients
- Teeth respond normally to pulp testing
- Patients are asymptomatic unless cyst becomes secondarily infected
- Can cause swelling and fluctuance of palatal tissues

Nasopalatine Duct Cyst (Incisive Canal Cyst)

- Occurs in the midline of the maxilla between central incisors
- Unilocular and well defined
- Usually no resorption of tooth structure

- Teeth respond normally to pulp testing
- Patients asymptomatic unless cyst becomes secondarily infected
- May cause swelling and inflammation of the incisive papillae

---

* * * * *   Clinical Note   * * * * *

The nasopalatine duct cyst is mistaken commonly for a
periradicular radiolucency of pulpal origin. Clinical tests
and proper angulation of periradicular films will aid in
making the correct diagnosis. The lesion, although able
to encompass the periradicular area of either central
incisor, will not cause widening of the periodontal
ligament space or dissolution of the lamina dura
around the central incisors. In addition, the
radiolucent lesion can be shifted off of
the root by using an angled film
for diagnosis.

Primordial Cyst

- Detected on routine radiographic series
- Patient usually unaware of its presence
- May be unilocular or multilocular
- Usually occurs as result of missing teeth
- Found at any age

Residual Cyst

- Cyst that remains after the extraction of a tooth
- Can occur anywhere in mouth
- Usually unilocular
- Usually does not increase in size
- Patients are asymptomatic
- Teeth respond normally to pulp testing

Scar Tissue

- Occurs in both the mandible and maxilla
- Can occur in all populations and at all ages
- Usually unilocular

- Occurs when a lesion of endodontic origin causes both lingual (palatal) and facial (buccal) cortical plates to be resorbed

- Persistent radiolucent "lesion" which does not resolve after endodontic treatment

- Occurs primarily after periradicular surgery and/or conventional endodontic treatment

- Often remains even after tooth is removed

★ ★ ★ ★ ★   Clinical Note   ★ ★ ★ ★ ★

Too often after root canal therapy, a persistent lesion is labeled as "apical scar tissue." The true apical scar is one of the more uncommon lesions (<2%) and yet is probably one of the most commonly used clinical terms to diagnose a persistent radio-lucency. In all probability the radiolucency that does not resolve completely after nonsurgical root canal therapy or after endodontic surgery is, histologically, the same tissue that was present before treatment (granuloma or cyst). Additional therapy is indicated.

Traumatic Bone Cyst

- Usually occurs in the mandible

- May be unilocular (most often) or multilocular

- Classically have "scalloped" borders that extend between the roots of teeth

- Seen in younger patients primarily

- Teeth respond normally to pulp testing

- Patients are asymptomatic unless cyst becomes secondarily infected

E. RADIOPAQUE LESIONS

Cementoma

- Most common in black middle-aged females; however, does occur in all populations and age groups

- Usually occurs in anterior mandibular teeth

- All teeth are responsive to pulp testing

- Early lesion(s) is radiolucent but becomes radiopaque over time (months to years)

- Usually multiple lesions are present

- Patients are asymptomatic

***** Clinical Note *****

The radiolucent lesions in Stage I of the cementoma do not cause loss of lamina dura or a widening of the periodontal ligament space routinely. This is one of the most important radiographic signs the clinician should note when differentiating these lesions from true lesions of pulpal origin.

Condensing Osteitis
(Chronic Focal Sclerosing Osteomyelitis)

- Occurs with all age groups
- Reaction of periradicular bone to chronic inflammation of pulp
- Can occur in any tooth; more commonly seen in mandibular molar and premolar regions
- Patient is asymptomatic unless pulp is acutely inflamed
- Teeth usually respond to pulp testing in early stages
- Some suggest radiopaque area resolves after pulpal inflammation is resolved

***** Clinical Note *****

The presence of condensing osteitis alone does not justify root canal treatment in the absence of irreversible symptoms and/or clinical tests. Often, very mild pulpal inflammation can cause condensing osteitis and conservative pulpal therapy will resolve the patient's symptoms without the need for additional endodontic treatment.

Fibrous Dysplasia

- Occurs in younger patients primarily
- Very slow growing lesion
- May occur as monostotic (fibrous dysplasia) or polyostotic (Albright's syndrome) form
- More frequently in maxilla
- Radiographic presentation is classical for "ground glass appearance"
- Patients are usually asymptomatic

Odontoma

- Unusual presentation of radiopacities composed of enamel, dentin, and cementum
- Can sometimes be associated with other lesions of odontogenic origin
- Occurs with all age groups
- Does not usually cause resorption of surrounding tooth structure

Ossifying Fibroma

- More common in young adults
- Can occur in both mandible and maxilla; however, primarily found in the posterior mandible
- Begin as radiolucencies and become calcified or cementified over time
- Very slow growing
- Patients are asymptomatic
- Often have expansion of the mandibular bone and displacement of teeth

Osteoblastoma (Cementoblastoma)

- Usually occurs in the mandibular posterior region
- Occurs in younger patients
- Closely related to the cementoblastoma
- Can cause resorption of tooth structure
- Does cause expansion of the bone
- Has characteristic radiolucent border around a radiopaque mass

Osteosarcoma

- Usually occurs in younger patients
- Mandible more commonly affected than maxilla
- Not uncommon for patients to have symptoms (pain, swelling, expansion of bone) similar to pulpal pathosis
- True malignant tumor
- Classical "sunburst" appearance of radiopaque lesion is uncommon

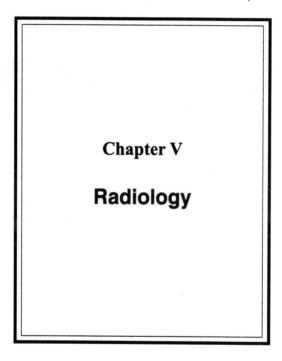

Chapter V

Radiology

RADIOLOGY

A. THE ENDODONTIC PRETREATMENT FILM AND BASIC ENDODONTIC RADIOGRAPHIC PRINCIPLES

- Always take a medical history before exposing any patient to radiographs
- Start film is only a 2-dimensional representation of a 3-dimensional object
- The start film is, perhaps, the most important film taken during endodontic therapy — can provide potentially the following information:
    - Justification or negation for treatment
    - Size of pulp chamber (2-dimension)
    - Number of canals
    - Number of roots
    - Curvature of roots
    - Presence of caries
    - Presence of periradicular pathosis
    - Presence of radicular pathosis (resorption, fracture, etc)
    - Dental history of a tooth
    - Periodontal status of a tooth
    - Level of calcification of the pulp chamber and canal system
    - Length of the roots
    - Method for assessing whether endodontic therapy was successful
- Along with the clinical presentation, this film can justify or negate the need for endodontic treatment
- If possible, obtain as many previous radiographs of tooth in question as possible before treating patient
- Start film may be digital or conventionally processed film

***** **Clinical Note** *****

Although controversial, the D speed films appear to provide a better quality film and are of more diagnostic value than E speed films.

- For diagnostic purposes, a periapical film should always be exposed

---

***** **Clinical Note** *****

Never rely on a film from another practitioner as the sole
source for diagnosis and interpretation of existing
pathosis. A new start film should always be
exposed regardless if treatment is anticipated.
This fact is even more critical if the
patient, prior to being referred,
has been treated previously.

- Bitewing, panorex, and/or occlusal films may be used as additional reference sources; however, they should never be the substitute for periapical films

---

***** **Clinical Note** *****

Maxillary pretreatment films exposed with a paralleling device
are sometimes at an angle which will prevent decay in the
crown from being clearly demonstrated. If it is suspected
that there is decay around a crown or large restoration, a bitewing film is indicated as an adjunct to
the periapical film to provide a better diagnostic
view of the coronal tooth structure.

- Should examine film for changes in both the coronal tooth structure and periapical architecture
- Paralleling device (eg, Rinn XCP-Rinn Corp, Elgin Illinois) should always be used to expose the start film

    – Provides greater likelihood of duplicating correct angle for subsequent recall films

    – Hemostats and similar film-holding devices should not be used for initial films as the best angle for proper diagnosis is difficult to achieve with these devices

- Provides best angle for radiographic interpretation of crown structures, pulp chamber, and root canal anatomy

---

***** **Clinical Note** *****

Exposing the patient to multiple-angled films is not essential
and is strongly discouraged as they do not provide
significant additional information required to
perform proper endodontic therapy.

- All sinus tracts should be traced with a size 25-35 gutta-percha cone prior to exposing the diagnostic pretreatment film

---

***** **Clinical Note** *****

Radiographic films are interpreted in various ways and, therefore, radiographs are subject to opinion and potential bias regarding the presence or absence of pathosis and/or potential radiographic changes from normal. Multiple factors can influence the ability to detect radiographic pathosis. Therefore, the more information about a tooth that can be obtained (from historical films providing different angulations, bitewings, etc), the more accurate the diagnosis will be.

- If the root canal system appears to be asymmetric to the long axis of the root, the clinician should suspect a second canal

  - Regardless of the angle at which a periapical film is exposed, if only one canal is present, it will be centered in the middle of the root

---

***** **Clinical Note** *****

An object that is positioned in the center of a root cannot be "moved" off of the center by manipulating the angulation of a film. However, an object that is "off center" can usually be moved onto the center of a root by changing the angulation of exposure. This factor is significant when determining the exact location of canals within multirooted teeth, perforations, broken instruments, etc.

- Angled films are extremely helpful in determining the presence or absence of one or more canals in a single root since, if only one canal is present, it will be positioned directly in the center of the root regardless of the angle of exposure

B. CONVENTIONAL VS DIGITAL RADIOGRAPHY

- Current exposure for conventional films, although extremely low, is significantly higher than that required by digital radiographs

- As of the writing of this Handbook, digital films are not significantly better for diagnosis of periapical pathosis than conventional films

- Digital radiographs are more convenient and significantly faster to produce and to process than conventional radiographs
- Must purchase at least one computer system for operatory
- Eliminates need for storage and categorization of radiographs
- Access to historical films is significantly faster than by conventional filing methods
- Storage capacities of current computer systems are sufficient for patient database

Digital Imaging

- Two-part process

    Sampling – Process used to digitize information about an image

    - Image divided into various sampling points called pixels (picture elements)
    - Greater the number of pixels, better the quality of digitized image

    Quantization – Process of digitizing the brightness information about an object

    - Range of the brightness scale is the gray scale
    - Greater the gray scale the closer the image is to its original
    - Humans can see thousands of shades of colors
    - Humans can only perceive about 30 shades of gray
- Uses a CCD (charged couple device) or PSP (photostimulable phosphor plate) system to capture the image
- Most video camcorders are CCD technology
- Hubble Space Telescope has same technology
- Two types of charged couple devices
    - Linear array (a scanning process)
    - Area array (periapical film technique)
- Charged Couple Devices
    - Made of high grade pure silicon
    - X-ray photons generate electron hole pairs to generate image

- – Can be used multiple times
- Photostimulable Phosphor Plates
    - – Uses a phosphor plate instead of film
    - – Exposed films must be scanned by a laser device
    - – Scanner converts light image into an electronic digital image
    - – First introduced in 1983
    - – In third generation
    - – Advantage over CCD systems is that with PSP there is a greater latitude of error with respect to exposure dose

Advantages of Digital Over Conventional Radiography

- Faster/instantaneous viewing of the radiograph after exposure
- Chemicals, wet tanks, or dark room not required
- Clinician has the opportunity to access patient records from any other location
- Clinician has the ability to manipulate radiographs and correct for exposure errors (under/over exposure)
- Images manipulated into simulated 3-D projections
- Images e-mailed to referring clinicians with other attachments and notes
- Images can be labeled with important information
- Excellent comparisons of historical films with recent films
- Systems (patient data bases, etc) networked within one office or among multiple offices
- Patient acceptance extremely high
- Patient education regarding endodontic procedure is more easily described and presented from CRT vs conventional film
- Ability to magnify specific areas of radiograph
- Ability to measure length of root for assessing working length estimations
- Standard of care for 2000s

Disadvantages of Digital Over Conventional Radiography

- Potential for fraudulent use
- Requires CPU in every operatory or portable laptop units

- If office is networked and network goes down, cannot access radiographs

- Expense of upgrading software programs, both digital radiography systems and operating systems

- Benefits of these systems outweigh greatly the few disadvantages

C. ASSESSING ENDODONTIC SUCCESS / RECALL

- Endodontic success rates range from 83% to 95%

- Can have clinical success, but radiographic failure

- Post treatment asymptomatic patients do not always correlate with radiographic resolution of lesion

- Minimum 6-month follow-up after completion of therapy if radiographic evidence of lesion at time of therapy

- Suggest 18- to 24-month follow-up if no lesion present at time of therapy to assure radiographic success of case

- Essential to have same angulation for final film as the recall film

- At recall visit, three potential radiographic scenarios if lesion was present at time of therapy:

  - Lesion is no longer radiographically discernible

  - Lesion is same size, slightly smaller, or slightly larger

  - Lesion is significantly smaller but still present

- Consider case unsuccessful if lesion is same size or slightly larger

- If lesion is only slightly smaller, high likelihood that case unsuccessful, but may, in absence of symptoms, wait additional 3-6 months

- If lesion is significantly smaller, suggest additional radiograph in 3-6 months

- Lesion should be significantly smaller at 6 months

***** **Clinical Note** *****

If the patient is asymptomatic after endodontic therapy but maintains a radiographic lesion of substantial size, additional therapy is warranted. It is highly unlikely that a lesion will resolve without additional treatment if 6 months after root canal therapy it still remains.

FREQUENTLY ASKED QUESTIONS (FAQs)

1. ***Do I need to purchase a digital radiography system?***

    The answer to this question is twofold. If you want to keep up with the state of the art technology in dentistry, then yes. Do you want to see better film quality, then no. There is not adequate scientific evidence that digital radiology technology will provide the practitioner with a better quality of diagnostic aids. With respect to patient education and acceptance, there is no better system to provide information about a patient's treatment plan.

2. ***What type of system should I purchase?***

    Because, as of the printing of this Handbook, there are only two systems available on the market, the choice is a function of convenience. The CCD system is more convenient than the PSP now; however, there is no quality difference with respect to the clinical level. Most systems are comparable. The best answer is to have at least two of the CCD and two PSP systems in your office for consignment purposes. Then after evaluating all four, select the one you feel most comfortable working with in the clinical situation.

3. ***Is it better to wait several months after root canal therapy before placing a permanent cast restoration on a tooth?***

    In the absence of complications during therapy, or if the patient is asymptomatic after completion of therapy, there is no justification for waiting some specific period of time before restoring the tooth. The main contraindication for immediately restoring a patient's tooth after root canal therapy is if the patient remains symptomatic. In these cases, permanent restorations will not resolve the patient's symptoms and will likely augment the problem.

Chapter VI

Armamentarium & Instruments in Nonsurgical Root Canal Treatment

ARMAMENTARIUM AND INSTRUMENTS IN NONSURGICAL ROOT CANAL TREATMENT

A. RUBBER DAM AND SUPPORTING MATERIALS

- The use of the rubber dam is mandatory during nonsurgical root canal treatment

- Facilitates treatment by isolating the tooth, preventing the inadvertent aspiration of small, endodontic instruments, preventing bacterial contamination during root canal treatment, protecting the oral, soft tissues, improving visibility and enhancing the efficiency of the dentist

Rubber Dam

- A thin, flat, sheet of latex of varying thickness and multiple colors

- Available in sizes of 5 X 5 or 6 X 6 inches

- Also available in nonlatex for those who may have demonstrated latex allergies

Rubber Dam Frame

- A plastic or metal device that retracts and stabilizes the rubber dam over the patient's mouth

Rubber Dam Clamp

- A metallic or plastic hook-like object, available in a variety of anatomical shapes, fits around the cervical portion of the tooth, retains and stabilizes the rubber dam

- Aids in soft tissue retraction immediately adjacent to the tooth

Rubber Dam Punch

- A metallic device used to place a small hole in the rubber dam so it will fit over the tooth

Rubber Dam Forceps

- A metallic pliers-type device that carries the rubber dam clamp and secures it around the tooth
- During placement of the clamp, the rubber dam may or may not be attached

B. DENTAL BURS FOR TOOTH ACCESS

- Access to the pulp chamber of the tooth is achieved by using rotary high-speed burs on a dental handpiece or turbine to gain entry through the lingual surface of the tooth (anterior teeth) or occlusal surface (posterior teeth)
- Many types of burs have been advocated and correct choice is based on tooth size and experience and skill

Burs

- Sizes 2, 4, and 6 round
- Long shank 556
- Safe ended diamonds
- Endo Z burs

C. INSTRUMENTS FOR PULP EXTIRPATION AND INITIAL CANAL DEBRIDEMENT

- Removal of the coronal portion of the pulp (pulpotomy) usually performed with a long shank spoon excavator or a rotary bur on a slow speed handpiece
- Removal of the dental pulp from the root canals (pulpectomy) or the necrotic pulp tissue (debridement) accomplished with many different instruments

Root Canal Broach

- A very narrow, round metallic instrument with barbs placed along its shaft
- The depth of entry into the pulp canal is limited by the size of the canal
- Used passively in the canal and should not engage dentin
- May also be used to remove necrotic debris and cotton products that may have been used in the chamber between treatments

Rotary Orifice Shaping Instrument

- A variable, tapered nickel titanium instrument used in a controlled speed, high torque handpiece
- Use in the canal is generally limited to the coronal half to two-thirds of the canal

D. IRRIGANTS AND CHELATING AGENTS IN NONSURGICAL ROOT CANAL TREATMENT

- Cleaning of the root canal system of its tissue, necrotic debris, bacteria, and toxins is accomplished with solutions designed to dissolve tissue and destroy bacteria
- Rinsing action during placement assists in thorough removal of the debris generated during the shaping of the root canal
- Serve as lubricants for the metallic instruments that are used in the canal
- Delivered to canal in a syringe with nonbinding, blunt-tipped needles
  - Needle tips should never be placed to the point of binding in the canal prior to delivery of irrigant

Sodium Hypochlorite

- Solution used in percentages from 1% to 5.25% to clean the root canal-known commonly as household bleach
- Dissolves tissue and kills bacteria rapidly – rinses and lubricates
- Rate of activity is related to the concentration
- Solution works best at 5.25%
  - As alternative, a 2.5% solution that is warmed to body temperature prior to use is highly effective

Hydrogen Peroxide

- Solution used in a 3% concentration
- Less effective than sodium hypochlorite and is not recommended as a routine irrigant
- May assist in stanching hemorrhage and often used alternately with sodium hypochlorite

EDTA (Ethylenediaminetetraacetic Acid)

- Chelating agent used in conjunction with sodium hypochlorite
- Used in liquid or paste form with special additives
- Paste enhances lubrication for metallic instruments
- Used usually in a 17% concentration of the active agent
- Assists in smear layer removal, softens the dentin, and may facilitate the loosening of calcific obstructions in the root canal

---

***** **Clinical Note** *****

The dictates for successful nonsurgical root canal treatment demand that the canal system be free of organic debris and that bacterial contamination be eliminated or minimized. Irrigation with solutions that enhance this goal is essential and, therefore, the use of water or saline for this purpose is contraindicated.

E. INSTRUMENTS FOR CLEANING AND SHAPING OF THE ROOT CANAL

- Special instruments are necessary for cleaning and shaping because of the unique and variable anatomy of root canal systems

Root Canal Files (K-Files)

- Long, thin, tapered metallic instruments made from rectangular, triangular or rhomboidal cross-sectional wires
- Instruments are stainless steel or nickel titanium and are created by either twisting or grinding
- Cutting angles on the wires are created that are used to scrape and clean the root canal
- Files are generally used in the root canal in a push-pull, twisting, watch-winding or circumferential motion within the canal
- The nature of the metal, the size of the instrument, and its cross-sectional configuration determine flexibility of each instrument
- Instruments are generally manufactured in lengths ranging from 21-31 mm

- The size of the instrument is determined by the diameter of the shaft 1.0 mm from the tip of the shaft and is recorded in decimal sizes based on mm dimensions
- Instruments have a standard taper of a 0.02 mm increase per mm increase up the shaft from the apical determining dimension
  - For example, a size 25 instrument has an apical dimension of 0.25 mm that increases to a dimension of 0.57 mm 16 mm up the shaft from the apical dimension.

Root Canal Files (Hedström Files)

- Long, thin, tapered metallic instruments made from round cross-sectional wires
- Stainless steel or nickel titanium and created by grinding cutting angles in its shaft
- Generally used in the root canal in a rasping, scraping motion as the file moves out of the canal
- Nature of the metal, size of the instrument, and its cross-sectional configuration determine flexibility of each instrument
- Generally manufactured in lengths ranging from 21-30 mm
- Size of the instrument determined by the diameter of the shaft 1.0 mm from the tip of the shaft and is recorded in decimal sizes based on mm dimensions
- Have a standard taper of a 0.02 mm increase per mm increase up the shaft from the apical determining dimension
  - For example, a size 25 instrument has an apical dimension of 0.25 mm that increases to a dimension of 0.57 mm 16 mm up the shaft from the apical dimension

Root Canal Files (Rotary Files)

- Long, thin, tapered metallic instruments made of nickel titanium and ground to create radial land cutting regions along the shaft
- Used in a rotary motion in the canal with consistent speed and high torque
- Have a variable taper of a 0.02, 0.04, or 0.06 mm increase per mm increase up the shaft from the apical determining dimension

Root Canal Reamers

- Long, thin, tapered metallic instruments made from rectangular, triangular, or rhomboidal cross-sectional wires
- Stainless steel and used by hand or in a rotary handpiece

- Instruments cut only in the in-stroke
- Have less cutting edges than a root canal file and less efficient
- Tend to deviate from the unique anatomy of the root canal system during its action
- Contemporary practices of endodontics do not favor or support its use in the cleaning and shaping of root canals

F. INSTRUMENTS FOR ROOT CANAL OBTURATION

- Consist primarily of sealer placing instruments, spreaders, and pluggers
- Spreaders and pluggers available in hand or finger-type instruments and made of either stainless steel or nickel titanium

Lentulo Spiral

- Twisted, corkscrew-shaped, metallic instrument designed specifically for the placement of root canal sealers

---

* * * * *   Clinical Note   * * * * *

These instruments must fit loosely in the canal and are not designed for active engagement of the dentin. If they bind or actively engage dentin, there is a high likelihood for breakage. The same instrument may be used by hand or in a rotary slow-speed handpiece.

Root Canal Spreader

- Long (17-29 mm), tapered, metallic instrument with a pointed tip
- Designed to fit within the prepared root canal and used to compact the gutta-percha filling material and sealer laterally against the root walls
- Provides a limited vertical component of compaction
- Available with a short plastic or metal handle that makes it look similar to a root canal file – known as a "finger spreader"

> ***** Clinical Note *****
>
> These instruments must fit loosely in the canal and are not designed for active wedging against the dentin walls. If they bind or actively engage dentin, there is a high likelihood that the root may crack or fracture. In order to be used effectively, they must penetrate the canal alongside the master gutta-percha cone to its apical extent.

Root Canal Plugger

- Long (18-29 mm), tapered, metallic instrument with a flattened or blunt tip

- Designed to fit within the prepared root canal and used to compact the gutta-percha filling material and sealer vertically to the apical extent of the canal preparation

- Also provides a lateral component of compaction

- Available with a short plastic or metal handle that makes it look similar to a root canal file – known as a "finger plugger"

> ***** Clinical Note *****
>
> These instruments must fit loosely in the canal and are not designed for active wedging against the dentin walls. If they bind or actively engage dentin, there is a high likelihood that the root may crack or fracture. In order to be used effectively, they must penetrate the canal freely to a point 3-5 mm from the apical extent of the prepared canal.

Other Instruments for Obturation

ROTARY COMPACTORS

- Used in electric or air driven slow speed hand pieces

- Rotation creates frictional heat and in-and-out action of the instrument is purported to compact gutta-percha filling material

ULTRASONIC TIPS

- Some ultrasonic units have tips that are recommended for the compaction of gutta-percha

G. ROOT CANAL SEALERS – CEMENTS

- Essential for complete root canal obturation
- Should be biocompatible and well tolerated by the periradicular tissues
- Mixed into a thick, creamy consistency
- Placed in root canal system with core gutta-percha filling material
- Most will set firm within a few minutes to hours
- Grouped as follows:
    - Zinc oxide-eugenol
    - Calcium hydroxide
    - Resins
    - Glass ionomers
    - Silicones

---

* * * * * Clinical Note * * * * *

The most commonly used sealers are zinc oxide-eugenol or
calcium hydroxide based. There are extensive studies
available that support their efficacy and safety.
A sealer from these choices is encouraged.

H. OBTURATION MATERIALS

- Historically, many materials have been used to fill the root canal space
- Must demonstrate minimal toxicity and tissue irritability
- Contemporary practice dictates the use of gutta-percha as the material of choice
    - Least allergenic obturating material available when retained within the root canal system

Paste-Filling Materials

- Not advocated for the filling of root canals

Silver Cones

- Historically, used to fill root canals

- Do not fulfill the contemporary tenets for a root canal filling material
- Their use is not recommended

Gutta-Percha

- Originally, the refined, coagulated milky exudate from certain trees indigenous to the Malayan Archipelago
- Presently used primarily in a synthetic form
- Can exist in different isomeric forms – an alpha and beta form
- Changes from alpha to beta at temperatures of 42°C to 44°C
- Changes into an amorphous melt at 56°C to 64°C
- During cooling to 37°C shrinkage occurs due to phase transformation to the beta state
- Alpha phase is subjected to less shrinkage
- Most contemporary gutta-percha used in a thermoplasticized state has been re-engineered into the alpha phase
- Can be softened with chemicals, such as chloroform
- Comes in multiple forms, such as cones and pellets
- Approximate composition of dental gutta-percha is 19% to 22% gutta-percha, 59% to 75% zinc oxide
    - Remaining small percentages a combination of waxes, coloring agents, antioxidants, and metallic salts
- Due to zinc oxide component, some antimicrobial activity is present
- For use in the root canal as a cone, both standardized and nonstandardized cones are available
- Must be used with a root canal sealer-cement
- Must be compacted to conform to the three-dimensional irregularities of the prepared root canal system

FREQUENTLY ASKED QUESTIONS (FAQs)

1. *Is it necessary to use a rubber dam during root canal treatment?*

    Use of the rubber dam is the "standard of care" when doing nonsurgical root canal treatment.

2. *If a tooth is fractured below the tissue level and a rubber dam cannot be placed, can the treatment be done without the dam?*

If a rubber dam cannot be readily placed on an individual tooth, other options are available: 1) clamp an adjacent tooth; 2) do a buildup on the tooth for purposes of clamping and isolation; 3) the tooth probably needs crown lengthening prior to root canal treatment – this will ensure success with the isolation and the ultimate tooth restoration.

3. *Don't rotary nickel-titanium instruments break easily in the canal?*

Not if they are used properly. Breakage occurs because of too much pressure, too much speed, choosing instruments too large for the canal anatomy, and failure to assess the nature of the canal anatomy, looking for curves, calcifications, and abrupt deviations.

4. *What is the best way to make an access opening in a porcelain or porcelain-fused to metal crown?*

Use a new, sharp, round diamond bur along with copious water spray on the high speed handpiece. Light pressure during cutting is necessary.

5. *Isn't hydrogen peroxide just as effective as sodium hydroxide when used as a canal irrigant?*

The two most important properties for an irrigant are its ability to kill or neutralize a wide range of bacteria and to dissolve tissue. Sodium hypochlorite is far superior to hydrogen peroxide in both regards.

6. *Would not a combination of hydrogen peroxide and sodium hypochlorite be more effective than either solution by itself?*

Ironically, the concomitant use of both solutions tends to negate their most important properties.

7. *Can sodium hypochlorite dissolve both necrotic and vital tissue effectively?*

Both tissues are dissolved and neutralized rapidly by sodium hypochlorite.

8. *There are clinical claims that sodium hypochlorite can cause pain and tissue destruction if it gets into the periradicular tissues. Is this true?*

If forced beyond the apex under pressure, it can cause these problems. The incidental passage of small amounts of sodium hypochlorite beyond the apical foramen during nonsurgical root canal treatment will cause no appreciable problems.

Chapter VII

Working Length Determination in Nonsurgical Endodontics

WORKING LENGTH DETERMINATION IN NONSURGICAL ENDODONTICS

DEFINITION

- Distance from a reproducible point on the coronal portion of the tooth to an identifiable point in the apical portion of the root

- Position is used for the apical extent of canal cleaning and shaping, and for the apical terminal placement of the root canal filling material

A. GENERAL CHARACTERISTICS AND ANATOMICAL CONSIDERATIONS

- Cemental-dentinal junction not used for this determination because it is a histological point that cannot be determined clinically

- Any point located apical to the cemental-dentinal junction would be considered to be in the surrounding periodontal ligament and inappropriate for the termination point of canal cleaning, shaping, and obturation

- Position of the working length should be in sound dentin, ideally at a point closely approximating the apical foramen

- Apical foramen usually exits from the canal anywhere from 0.5-2.0 mm or more coronally and, oftentimes, laterally to the root apex

- If apical resorption is present or if there is a radiolucency at the root apex, the canal may exit even farther from the position stated above

- Tactile sensation not recommended on a regular basis for determining working length because multiple variations exist in the apical anatomy of the root canal

- Apical variations may influence working length determination

  - Accessory canals, canal splitting, an apical delta, apical calcification, apical blockage, variations in the position and nature of the cemental-dentinal junction, and apical resorption

- Radiographs commonly used to determine this position

- Electronic apex locators also used

B. CLINICAL TECHNIQUE WITH RADIOGRAPHS

- Good preoperative radiograph essential
- Length of the tooth estimated from this radiograph
- Size, shape, position, and curvature of the root should be noted
- Approximately 1 mm is subtracted from the estimated working length and an appropriately sized root canal file teased to this length within the canal
    - Expose radiograph (see Chapters IV and V)
- Two radiographs may be used in multi-rooted teeth
    - One taken from a straight-on view and one from an angled view
    - Allows for the separation of closely approximated roots or canals

---

***** **Clinical Note** *****

Application of the buccal object rule essential. If the radiograph(s) show that the file is >1 mm shorter or longer than the desired position, an interpolation of variance is made, the original estimate is corrected, and a new set of radiographs are exposed to verify the proper working length.

***** **Clinical Note** *****

If >1 mm from the desired working length, additional radiographs are required to assure accurate length determination.

- If length is within 1 mm of the desired location, a clinical correction is made and noted as the adjusted or final working length
- Gross anatomical variations that may interfere with working length
    - Exostoses, zygomatic process, severe root anagulation, and root overlapping
- Radiographic determination of working length only provides a two-dimensional assessment of such and a suggestion of further variations in a third-dimension

```
* * * * *   Clinical Note   * * * * *
The coronal position chosen for determining the working length
must be on sound tooth structure. For example, in anterior
teeth the incisal edge is preferred. In posterior teeth, a
sound cusp tip is oftentimes used. The reference
point must be noted in the record along with
the recording of the working for each canal.
Consistency in documentation
is essential.
```

C. GUIDELINES FOR TAKING RADIOGRAPHS WITH DIFFERENT TOOTH GROUPS

- The buccal object rule is essential to separate roots or canals in teeth with roots that are wide buccolingually
- Can be used in either a mesiodistal format or anterior-superior format

Maxillary Teeth

- Anterior teeth usually taken from a straight view
- Lateral incisors and canines require special attention because of palatal, distal curvatures and length, respectively
- Premolars are usually viewed from the mesial, thereby splitting the two roots or canals on the radiograph
    - Some cases may warrant a distal view radiograph
- Molars are usually viewed from the buccal
    - If a second canal is suspected in the mesiobuccal root, a distal view is recommended

Mandibular Teeth

- Anterior teeth often require multiple views to detect the multitude of canal variations
- Premolars can be viewed straight on, as the presence of the extra canals is usually in the mesiodistal view
    - Occasionally, a mesial view is required
- Molars are usually viewed both straight on and from the mesial
    - The latter radiographic view permits separation of the mesiobuccal root canal from the mesiolingual root canal
    - Can also determine the presence of multiple canals in the distal root

    –   Occasionally a distal view radiograph is required for mandibular molars

D. CLINICAL TECHNIQUE WITH APEX LOCATORS

- Used in a resistance type, impedance type, or frequency type of electrical format

- Errors can occur with all types of units, due to fluid in the canal, improper contacts, presence of canal variations, and so forth

- Dry canals are essential with resistance type locators

- Impedance type must be calibrated and may demonstrate problems in young or immature teeth

- Frequency type can operate in a canal filled with pus and tissue; however, filling of the entire chamber with an electroconductive solution is to be avoided

- Contact with coronal restorations must be avoided with all types

- Ideally, the measuring probe or file should be inserted partially into the canal prior to attaching the leads from the locator power source

- Probe or file should fit canal snugly in all cases

- Often the working length must still be verified with a radiograph

- When possible, estimate the working length from the preoperative radiograph

- Tease the measuring probe or file part way into the canal and attach the electronic lead

- Oscillate the file back and forth while slowly advancing the file towards the apex

- As the file approaches the apex, the electric impedance or resistance changes and the position of the file is visualized on the units screen indicating that the file is within the canal or beyond

- Repeat this action multiple times to verify this desired position and length

    –   If verifiable, record it as the working length

> ***** **Clinical Note** *****
>
> With the availability of nickel titanium rotary endodontic orifice shapers and files to clean and shape the coronal portion of the canal (crown down technique), it is now easier to determine the working length with all techniques. Coronal interferences are eliminated with the crown down preparation technique. Therefore, the crown down approach to canal cleaning and shaping is recommended in the coronal 2/3 of the root canal prior to taking a working length determination with either technique described (see Chapter VIII).

FREQUENTLY ASKED QUESTIONS (FAQs)

1. ***Are electronic apex locators (EAL) a good replacement for dental radiographs used for working length determination?***

    While their performance and consistency have been enhanced, EALs cannot replace the dental radiograph. The dental radiograph provides a greater amount of information over and above the length of the tooth/the apical extent of the canal. EALs should be used to supplement the information gleaned from the radiograph.

2. ***What is the best type of apex locator?***

    Frequency-type EALs are most reliable and valid.

Chapter VIII

Cleaning & Shaping of the Root Canal System

CLEANING & SHAPING OF THE ROOT CANAL SYSTEM

- Cleaning and shaping (C&S) of the root canal system is considered paramount to successful root canal treatment

- Heretofore known as biomechanical and chemomechanical instrumentation, this process has the following goals:

    - Removal of all tissue debris, antigenic substrates, bacteria, bacterial toxins, predentin, and contaminated dentin

    - Disinfection of the root canal system

    - Creation of a specific cavity form in the canal to enhance its three-dimensional obturation

    - Creation of a continuously tapered funnel preparation from the apical extent of the canal (working length) to the coronal orifice essential

- Straight-line access to the root canal system necessary for thorough C&S

- Access openings placed routinely in the lingual surfaces of anterior teeth and the occlusal surfaces of posterior teeth

- Coronal portion of the canal often opened to a larger size with Gates Glidden burs or Orifice Shapers (see Chapter VI)

    - In large, straight canal, Peeso Reamers sometimes used

    - Use should be avoided in small, curved canals

- Instruments for root canal C&S (see Chapter VI) used in different motions or manners to facilitate achievement of the stated goals

- Motions include a filing or push-pull motion, a reaming or clockwise motion, a watch-winding or a left-right pulling motion, a balanced force or left-right pushing motion, or rotary planing motion

- Motions can be used in any given canal based on canal anatomy, clinician choice, and expertise

- Can be used in the center of the canal or around the walls (circumferential)

- Curved hand instruments in the apical 1-3 mm prior to insertion into the root canal (precurving)

- Cutting pressure on the instrument (hand) applied away from the inside of curve so that shaping occurs to the outer wall (anticurvature filing)

- Smaller file placed to the canal working length on a regular basis to remove any accumulated debris (recapitulation)

- Recapitulate prior to canal obturation to insure patency of canal to working length

- Routine passage of a small file beyond the working length during C&S to ensure that the apical foramen is open has been suggested (patency filing)

  - While used by some clinicians, there are no scientific data to support its practice

- All C&S are done with the root canal filled with irrigants and/or chelating agents

- Avoid C&S in dry canal

A. TECHNIQUES FOR C&S

- Generally, techniques for C&S can be placed in two categories with multiple variations within each — step back and crown down techniques

B. STEP BACK TECHNIQUE (telescopic technique, apical to coronal technique, passive step back technique)

- Refers to establishment of the working length immediately after access opening preparation

- Followed by the incremental enlargement, cleaning and shaping of the apical portion of the canal to a specific sized root canal instrument

- Subsequent enlargement of the middle and coronal portion of the canal by using progressively larger instruments short of the apical preparation

- Generally done by reducing the length of the file used in the canal by increments of 0.5-1.0 mm

  - For example: If the canal working length is 22.0 mm at a size #30 K-file, the next instrument used would be a size #35 K-file at 21.5 or 21.0 mm; followed by a size #40 K-file at 20.5 or 20.0 mm, and so forth until canal is shaped to a continuously tapered funnel preparation from the apical extent to the coronal orifice

Variations in the Step Back Technique

- Varying the length reduction of subsequent files between 0.5-2.0 mm when shaping from the apical to coronal portion of the canal

- Opening the coronal portion of the canal before working length determination

- Opening the coronal and middle portions before working length determination using either hand or rotary files

- Use of hedström files to do the step back shaping of the canal

- Following the step back technique, a crown down technique with hand or rotary instruments is used to smooth canal walls

C. CROWN DOWN TECHNIQUE (step down technique, balanced force, crown down pressureless technique)

- Orifice shapers, Gates Glidden burs, or hand instruments are used to open the coronal portion of the canal

- Action of the instruments is primarily rotational

- If hand instruments are used, reamers may be appropriate

- In most canals, tapered rotary instruments are more efficient and create the desired shape for the final canal preparation

- Subsequently, any of these same instruments, only smaller in size, may be used in the middle and coronal portion of the apical third of the canal

- Once the coronal 2/3 to 3/4 of the canal have been shaped in this manner, the working length is determined

- Continue cleaning and shaping using larger instruments, either hand or rotary, in the crown down manner to the apical constriction or in the apical 1.0-2.0 mm

- Choice of technique based on canal curvature, canal size, and degree of calcification

  - For example: Use a .07 tapered rotary orifice shaper in the coronal 2.0-3.0 mm

  - This is followed by a .06 and .05 tapered orifice shaper to the middle portion of the canal

  - Subsequently a .06 or .04 variable tapered instrument is used in the next few millimeters, followed by a .04 or .02 tapered rotary or hand instrument, thereby creating a continuously tapered funnel

Variations in the Crown Down Technique

- Use of the balanced force technique in which hand instruments are applied in a crown down manner, applying force in counter-clockwise and clockwise directions

- Shaping the coronal half of the canal with rotary instruments followed by hand instruments to open the apical half of the canal

- Integrated options from both the crown down and step back techniques to manage canals with extreme curvature, irregularities, or calcification

- Extensive use of Gates Glidden burs at various depths in the canal to create rapid access to the apical constriction

- Integration of Orifice Shapers with hand instruments to achieve the funneled shape

- Use of crown down followed by step back (double-flared technique)

D. PROBLEMS OCCURRING DURING C&S

- Multiple problems can occur during canal C&S

- Some are unique to the technique being used – hand (H) or rotary (R), step back (SB), or crown down (CD)

- Each error is identified and related to the technique identified

Canal Blockage
(H), (SB), (rarely CD)

- Results from tissue packing, debris accumulation, wall perforation, instrument separation, failure to use copious irrigation, rapid use of larger instrument sizes

Instrument Separation
(H), (R), (SB), (CD)

- Results from excessive stress or pressure, use of too large an instrument in a small canal, forcing of instruments that bind, excessive rotation speeds, failure to observe instrument flaws, excessive rotation of hand instruments

Ledges
(H), (SB), (R)

- Results from deviation from canal space

- Occurs with rotary instruments if large instruments used prematurely or if instruments (H) are not flexible or are forced apically

Perforations
(H), (R), (SB), (CD)

- Results from uncontrolled movement of the instrument in the canal after blocking or ledging; excessive use of large instruments in thin roots (strip); passage of large instruments beyond the root apex, thereby straightening the canal (zip or rip)

E. MANAGEMENT OF CHAMBER & ROOT PERFORATIONS

- Perforations must be identified as soon as possible
- Prevent contamination or irritation in site of perforation
- Control hemorrhage with sterile cotton and pressure
- Use minimal hemostatic agent if desired
- Seal immediately
- Seal chamber perforation with MTA – cover with glass ionomer
- Seal root perforation with MTA – possibly fill entire canal with agent
- Use minimal compaction during placement to minimize extrusion beyond tooth
- Other less desirable sealing agents – glass ionomer, zinc oxide-eugenol, amalgam, calcium hydroxide, and acid-etched composite
- May have to consider surgery – see Chapter XXI

Loss of Canal Length
(H), (R), (SB), (CD)

- Results from blockage, ledges, separated instruments, failure to observe reference points during C&S, use of stiff nonflexible instruments around canal curves

Overinstrumentation
(H), (R), (SB), (CD)

- Results from improper working length determination, failure to observe reference points during C&S, failure to recognize apical resorption

Overpreparation
(H), (R), (SB), (CD)

- Results from use of too many instruments for too long a time in the canal, use of instruments that are too large for the thin roots

Underpreparation
(H), (SB)

- Results from failure to shape canal in middle and coronal portions

F. MANAGEMENT OF THE SMEAR LAYER IN C&S

- The smear layer is formed on the walls of the root canal during canal C&S with hand and rotary instruments
- Layer may be even thicker with rotary instruments
- Layer consists of dentin chips, pulp tissue debris, and bacteria and their products
- Removal of this layer essential to achieve complete canal debridement and disinfection
- Can be accomplished in the following ways:
  - Use of chelating agents (EDTA) during the C&S (see Chapter VI)
  - Chelating agents used as liquids are highly effective
  - Upon completion of canal shaping, soak the canal for at least 60 seconds with liquid EDTA (can be done for up to 2 minutes)
    - Rinse the canal thoroughly with sodium hypochlorite and dry with paper points
    - Obturate the canal

***** Clinical Note *****

Concern has been expressed by some clinicians that the EDTA and sodium hypochlorite may be weakening the root dentin through excessive demineralization. This has not been shown scientifically and is viewed only as an empirical concern at this point.

FREQUENTLY ASKED QUESTIONS (FAQs)

1. *Is rotary instrumentation better than hand instrumentation?*

    In the majority of root canal treatments, the use of both hand and rotary instruments is necessary to achieve the desired goals. However, rotary instruments appear to be more effective in rapid shaping and removal of debris from the canal system. They also create a canal shape that is more desirable and reproducible.

Chapter IX

Obturation of the Prepared Root Canal System

OBTURATION OF THE PREPARED ROOT CANAL SYSTEM

A. GOALS OF CANAL OBTURATION

- Eliminate all avenues of leakage from the oral cavity or the periradicular tissues into the root canal system
- Seal within the system, the irritants that cannot be removed fully during canal cleaning and shaping

B. CHARACTERISTICS OF AN IDEAL ROOT CANAL FILLING – STANDARD OF CARE

- Three-dimensional obturation of the entire root canal – no voids
- Positioned as close as possible to the apical constriction (histologically, the cemental-dentinal junction)
- Filled with gutta-percha and sealer
- Radiographic appearance of a dense filling
- Avoidance of gross overextension into the periradicular tissues
- No underfillings in the presence of a patent canal
- Use of paraformaldehyde-containing materials for obturation are below the standard of care

C. CRITERIA TO DETERMINE WHEN THE CANAL IS READY FOR OBTURATION

- Tooth isolated to prevent contamination during obturation
- Canal cleaned and shaped in a manner that will not compromise the obturation technique
- Canal clean and dry – absence of pus, blood, tissue fluids, and saliva
- All compacting instruments prefit to ensure proper depth of penetration in different parts of the canal – based on obturation technique
- Patient reasonably free of symptoms

```
* * * * *   Clinical Note   * * * * *

If the patient is still in pain or the original symptoms have not
  abated, obturation of the root canal system will not resolve
  the patient's symptoms. Do not consider obturation unless
     there is significant evidence that instrumentation of the
        root canal system has resolved the patients symptoms
           or that the symptoms are waning significantly.
```

D. OBTURATION TECHNIQUES

- Cold compaction of gutta-percha
- Compaction of gutta-percha softened in the canal and cold compacted
- Compaction of gutta-percha – thermoplasticized, injected into the system, and cold compacted
- Compaction of gutta-percha placed into the canal and softened mechanically
- Core-carrier techniques for delivery and compaction of gutta-percha

Cold Compaction

- Choose master gutta-percha cone that corresponds to final size of root canal instrument that passed freely to the working length
- Cone should fit with slight resistance to removal – referred to as "tugback"
- Select root canal spreader (hand or finger – see Chapter VI) that will penetrate alongside the master cone to working length or within 1.0 mm of it
- Place root canal sealer mixed to creamy consistency into the canal – attempt to coat the walls throughout the entire length of the canal
- Place master cone coated lightly with sealer
- Root canal spreader placed alongside cone and gutta-percha compacted both laterally and vertically
- Space created by spreader filled with additional gutta-percha cones – accessory cones – smaller in size and taper than master cone
- When spreader cannot penetrate more than 2-3 mm into canal orifice, compaction is complete
- Remove cones extending from the canal orifice with heat and compact vertically with plugger at the canal orifice

- Clean pulp chamber of gutta-percha and sealer

- Place sound temporary restoration or proceed immediately to permanent restoration

- Radiograph without rubber dam in place to determine adequacy of obturation

- Variations in technique

  – Apical adaptation of master cone with solvent or heat

  – Cold compaction only in apical third followed by compaction of warmed or thermoplasticized gutta-percha in the remainder of canal

Compaction of Gutta-Percha Softened in the Canal and Cold Compacted

- Choose a master gutta-percha cone that approximates the length and shape of the prepared canal

- Fit cone snuggly to within 1-2 mm of the working length

- Prefit various root canal pluggers (see Chapter VI) to different depths in the canal

- Place root canal sealer mixed to creamy consistency into the canal – attempt to coat the walls only in the position of the master cone – short of the working length

- Place master cone coated lightly with sealer slowly into canal – avoids pooling of sealer at apical extent of canal

- Use heated instrument to sear off coronal portion of gutta-percha cone – also transfers heat to remainder of cone

- Use cold vertical plugger to compact the gutta-percha apically and laterally

- Reapply heated instrument to remove additional 1-3 mm segments of gutta-percha apically followed by compaction with appropriately sized pluggers

- Ultimately the apical 2-3 mm of gutta-percha is delivered in a softened state into the prepared apical portion of the canal

- Expose radiograph to assess quality of apical obturation

- Add small (2-3 mm) segments of heat-softened gutta-percha into the canal and compact after each addition – obturates the coronal portion of the canal

- Clean pulp chamber of gutta-percha and sealer

- Place sound temporary restoration or proceed immediately to permanent restoration

- Radiograph without rubber dam in place to determine adequacy of obturation

- Variations in technique

  - Enhanced systems to control heat delivery to the gutta-percha (System B, Touch 'N Heat)

  - Injectable gutta-percha to fill the coronal portion after apical compaction (Obtura)

  - Thermocompaction of coronal portion with rotary instruments (JS Quick-fill)

Compaction of Gutta-Percha – Thermoplasticized, Injected into the System, and Cold Compacted

- Ensure canal shaped to continuously tapered funnel preparation for the apical extent to the canal orifice

- Prefit injection needle into canal to ensure depth of placement (3-5 mm from apical extent)

- Make sure needle does not bind at ideal depth

- Place new pellet of gutta-percha into heating chamber

- Place sealer on canal walls only to depth of injection needle placement

- Insert needle and inject slowly – permit build-up of injected material in canal to lift needle from canal

- Fill apical 1/2 of canal – compact with plugger

- Add additional portions of gutta-percha as necessary and compact

- Clean pulp chamber of gutta-percha and sealer

- Place sound temporary restoration or proceed immediately to permanent restoration

- Radiograph without rubber dam in place to determine adequacy of obturation

- Variations in technique

  - Fill entire canal – compact

  - Fill apical 2-3 mm with gutta-percha – compact

  - Fill only to level of anticipated post space preparation – compact

Compaction of Gutta-Percha Placed Into the Canal and Softened Mechanically

- Fit master cone as with cold compaction (above)
- Place sealer
- Seat cone with sealer
- Place rotating compactor adjacent to cone with gentle pressure to a point 3-4 mm short of the working length or until resistance met
- Hold compactor in position for 2-3 seconds
- Remove compactor while still rotating
- In wide canals, can use two or more gutta-percha cones
- Following removal of rotating instrument, additional cones or gutta-percha segments may be added and compacted
- Clean pulp chamber of gutta-percha and sealer
- Place sound temporary restoration or proceed immediately to permanent restoration
- Radiograph without rubber dam in place to determine adequacy of obturation

Core Carrier Techniques for Delivery and Compaction of Gutta-Percha

- Size and shape of canal is verified and correlated with size of core-carrier chosen
- Core-carrier is heated in special oven
- Sealer is placed in coronal 1/2 to 3/4 of canal
- Remove heated core-carrier from oven and place into canal slowly – minimal pressure to desired length
- Do not twist core-carrier during placement
- Verify radiographically if necessary
- Cut core-carrier slightly above orifice with rotating bur
- Place additional gutta-percha cones and compact if canal large in buccolingual direction
- Clean pulp chamber of gutta-percha and sealer
- Place sound temporary restoration or proceed immediately to permanent restoration
- Radiograph without rubber dam in place to determine adequacy of obturation

Radiographic Assessment of Canal Obturation

- Obturated canal should reflect shape that is approximately the same as the root morphology
- Obturated canal should be continuously tapered funnel shape
- Gutta-percha should be uniformly dense throughout the canal with absence of voids, gaps, and irregularities
- Gutta-percha and sealer retained within the confines of the root

FREQUENTLY ASKED QUESTIONS (FAQs)

1. *Why can't the canal be filled with a paste filling?*

    Paste filling cannot be compacted and, therefore, three-dimensional obturation is all but impossible. Pastes can break down easily in fluids and cannot be retained in the canal easily. Most pastes are toxic once they begin to undergo dissolution.

2. *Can root canals be retreated with the currently advocated obturation techniques?*

    Yes — these techniques can all be reversed. However, when cleaning and shaping and obturating canals, it should be done with the intent of "not having to retreat them."

3. *What is the best obturation technique?*

    All techniques are good. The ability to achieve success with all of them is, however, dependent on the quality of the canal clean and shaping – and the ultimate restoration that is placed on the tooth.

4. *Does gutta-percha have to be heated to use it successfully?*

    No — cold compaction of gutta-percha is very successful and has been used for decades as an obturation technique.

5. *I've had trouble using the core-carrier techniques and many have to be retreated – what is the problem?*

    The main reason for problems with core-carrier obturation techniques is lack of proper canal shaping. Use of the newer variable tapered nickel-titanium instruments for preparation creates ideal shapes for the use of the core-carrier techniques.

Chapter X

Local Anesthetics and Anesthetic Techniques

LOCAL ANESTHETICS AND ANESTHETIC TECHNIQUES

A. TYPES

- Esters and amides

- Esters are no longer in favor because of higher side effects and greater probability of allergic reactions

- Difficult to obtain dental local anesthetic ester types in U.S.

- Selection of local anesthetic should depend upon several factors

  - Desired length of duration of anesthesia

  - Procedure type (surgery, emergency treatment of "hot tooth," root canal treatment, etc)

  - Medical status of patient

  - Pulpal and periradicular diagnosis

B. MECHANISM OF ACTION

- Local anesthetics exhibit both a charged and uncharged form

  - Charged form is cation (positive charge)

  - Uncharged form is anion

- Ratio of charged and uncharged is a function of pH of both anesthetic and soft tissue and pKa of anesthetic

- Uncharged form passes through nerve sheath more readily because it is more lipid soluble

- After entering the nerve fiber, the anion dissociates again and the newly dissociated cations bind inside the sodium channel

- Areas of inflammation and purulence have a negative effect on local anesthetics because there are less anions to penetrate the nerve sheath and, subsequently, less dissociation into cations within the nerve

> ***** **Clinical Note** *****
>
> The inability to obtain profound anesthesia in the absence of
> purulence and other similar factors in the presence of a
> "hot tooth" have not been explained adequately. Block
> techniques proximal to the inflamed pulp are not
> sufficient to obtain profound anesthesia in many
> cases. Intrapulpal injections are often the only
> method by which adequate anesthesia
> can be obtained in many instances.

- Most local anesthetics have an onset of action between 1 and 20 minutes

C. NOMENCLATURE OF LOCAL ANESTHETICS

Short Duration Local Anesthetics (<60 minutes)

- 2% Lidocaine (Xylocaine®, Dilocaine®, Octocaine®, Nervocaine®)
- 3% Mepivacaine (Carbocaine® 3%, Isocaine® 3%, Polocaine® 3%)
- 4% Prilocaine (Citanest® 4%)

Moderate Duration Local Anesthetics (60-120 minutes)

- 2% Lidocaine w 1:50,000 or 1:100,000 epi (Octocaine® 50, Octocaine® 100, Xylocaine® w epi 1:100,000, 1:50,000)
- 2% Mepivacaine w 1:20,000 levonordefrin (Carbocaine® 2% w Neo-Cobefrin®, Isocaine® 2%, Polocaine® 2%)
- 4% Prilocaine w 1:200,000 epi (Citanest Forte® w epi)

Long Duration Local Anesthetics (>120 minutes)

- 0.5% Bupivacaine w 1:200,000 epi (Marcaine® w epi, Sensorcaine®)
- 1.5% Etidocaine w 1:200,000 epi (Duranest®)

D. COMMONLY USED LOCAL ANESTHETICS

2% Lidocaine w 1:50,000 or 1:100,000 epi (Octocaine® 50, Octocaine® 100, Xylocaine® w epi 1:100,000, 1:50,000)

- Amide type of local anesthetic
- Derivative of xylidine
- Available in 1.8 mL dental anesthetic carpules

- Usual dosage in adults is 0.9-3.6 mL

- Each carpule contains 36 mg of anesthetic, maximum dose is 8 carpules

- 2% Lidocaine w 1:100,000 epi used primarily for most endodontic procedures and routine dental work

- 2% Lidocaine w 1:50,000 epi usually reserved for use as a local injection into soft tissue in a surgical site for more efficient hemostasis during surgical procedures

- Detoxified primarily in liver

  − Should be used with caution in patients with severe liver disease

- Not contraindicated in patients with heart disease; however, dosage should be monitored closely

- 2% Lidocaine w 1:50,000 epi is not indicated for routine use as a mandibular block anesthetic

- Because of epinephrine content, should not be used routinely in patients on MAO inhibitors or tricyclic antide-pressants

- Not contraindicated in pregnant women (after 1st trimester) or in nursing mothers

3% Mepivacaine (Carbocaine® 3%, Isocaine® 3%, Polocaine® 3%) and 2% **Mepivacaine w 1:20,000 levonordefrin** (Carbocaine® 2% w Neo-Cobefrin®, Isocaine® 2%, Polocaine® 2%)

- Amide type of local anesthetic

- Derivative of xylidine

- Available in 1.8 mL dental anesthetic carpules (each carpule of 3% Mepivacaine contains 54 mg of anesthetic)

- Usual dosage in adults is 1.8-9 mL (maximum of 5 carpules of 3%)

- 3% Mepivacaine without vasoconstrictor is not indicated for routine endodontic procedures, as duration is usually too short

- High blood level concentrations of Mepivacaine may result CNS disturbances (eg, anxiety, dizziness, tremors, confu-sion)

- Have approximately same toxicity levels as xylocaine

- Because of levonordefrin content, should not routinely be used in patients on MAO inhibitors or tricyclic antidepres-sants

```
* * * * *    Clinical Note    * * * * *
Mepivacaine w levonordefrin does not provide clinically the
same level of anesthesia in routine endodontic procedures
as does lidocaine hydrochloride w epinephrine. Its use
during endodontic surgical procedures should be
avoided if hemostasis is a major concern.
```

4% Prilocaine (Citanest® Plain 4%) and **4% Prilocaine w 1:200,000 epi** (Citanest Forte® w epi)

- Amide type of local anesthetic
- Derivative of toluidine
- Available in 1.8 mL dental anesthetic carpules (each carpule contains 72 mg of anesthetic)
- Usual dosage in adults is 1.8-5.4 mL
- Maximum dose should not exceed 5 carpules
- Because of epinephrine content (Prilocaine w 1:200,000 epi), should not routinely be used in patients on MAO inhibitors or tricyclic antidepressants
- High blood level concentrations of Prilocaine may result in CNS disturbances (eg, anxiety, dizziness, tremors, confusion)

0.5% Bupivacaine w 1:200,000 epi (Marcaine® w epi, Sensorcaine®)

- Amide type of local anesthetic
- Derivative of xylidine
- Available in 1.8 mL dental anesthetic carpules (each carpule contains 9 mg of anesthetic)
- Maximum dosage is 10 carpules or about 90 mg of anesthetic
- Generally 2-3 times longer duration then xylocaine
- May provide anesthesia for 10-12 hours; however, usually a 5- to 7-hour range is normal
- Used generally as a local anesthetic for surgical procedures in endodontics and oral surgery because of the extended duration
- Because of epinephrine content (Bupivacaine w 1:200,000 epi), should not be used routinely in patients on MAO inhibitors or tricyclic antidepressants
- High blood level concentrations of Bupivacaine may result CNS disturbances (eg, anxiety, dizziness, tremors, confusion)

1.5% Etidocaine w 1:200,000 epi (Duranest®)

- Amide type of local anesthetic
- Derivative of xylidine
- Available in 1.8 mL dental anesthetic carpules (each carpule contains 27 mg of anesthetic)
- Usual dose is 1-2 carpules
- Maximum adult dosage is 8 carpules
- May provide anesthesia for 8-12 hours; however, usually a 5- to 8-hour range is normal
- Used generally as a local anesthetic for surgical procedures in endodontics and oral surgery because of the extended duration
- Because of epinephrine content (Etidocaine w 1:200,000 epi), should not routinely be used in patients on MAO inhibitors or tricyclic antidepressants
- High blood level concentrations of Etidocaine may result CNS disturbances (eg, anxiety, dizziness, tremors, confusion)

E. COMMONLY USED ANESTHETIC TECHNIQUES

Maxillary Anterior and Premolar Teeth

- For maxillary incisors, anesthetic should be deposited in the infraorbital region of the maxilla usually between the maxillary lateral and central incisors
- Short 25 g or 27 g needle is required for this technique
- This technique anesthetizes all anterior teeth on ipsilateral side and the premolar teeth if a maxillary anterior superior nerve block is achieved

---

***** Clinical Note *****

When performing root canal therapy on maxillary canine teeth, because of their excessive length (often 23-31 mm WLs), it is advisable to inject anesthetic directly over the apex of these teeth. In most cases, a full carpule of anesthetic (1.8 mL) will be sufficient to obtain profound anesthesia in the maxillary canine. Occasionally, palatal infiltration is required; however, it is not necessary to perform this procedure on a routine basis.

- In most cases, buccal infiltration or an anterior superior alveolar nerve block will provide profound anesthesia for the incisor teeth

---

***** **Clinical Note** *****

Maxillary lateral incisors occasionally demonstrate a palatal dilaceration that requires additional palatal infiltration of anesthetic. However, this is uncommon and is not required in most instances.

- Palatal infiltration is not usually indicated for root canal treatment of the maxillary incisors or canine teeth except when the rubber dam clamp impinges on the palatal tissue

---

***** **Clinical Note** *****

It is not necessary to give routinely an anterior palatine nerve block when performing root canal treatment on anterior teeth. This injection is usually reserved for surgical treatment in this area.

***** **Clinical Note** *****

When clamping maxillary anterior teeth, a premolar clamp is often more easily positioned and better seated than anterior rubber dam clamps. An ivory "0" or "00" premolar clamp will allow seating of the clamp without the need for additional anesthesia on the palatal tissues. Anterior clamps (#9, #212) are often too large and too difficult to manage properly in lieu of smaller premolar clamps. Anterior clamps should be used when a severe amount of tooth structure has been lost from an anterior tooth and there is little coronal structure remaining to be clamped.

- In most clinical situations, high buccal infiltration directly adjacent to the apex of a premolar tooth will provide profound anesthesia

- Maxillary first premolars will require palatal infiltration adjacent to the palatal root apex when performing root canal therapy

- Maxillary second premolars do not require palatal infiltration on a routine basis

Maxillary Molar Teeth

- When performing root canal treatment on maxillary first and second molars, both buccal and palatal anesthesia is required

- A posterior superior nerve block can be achieved by injecting anesthetic into the pterygomaxillary space

- Aspiration is critical with this injection because of the highly vascular plexus in this area

- A posterior superior nerve block will anesthetize routinely the maxillary second and third molar buccal roots

- The maxillary first molar will often require an additional infiltration over the mesiobuccal root as the middle superior alveolar nerve innervates this root in greater than one-quarter of the population.

---

* * * * *   Clinical Note   * * * * *

In most instances, the buccal roots of all maxillary molars can be anesthetized by infiltration techniques directly into the buccal mucosa adjacent to the apex of the buccal roots. Often, only one carpule of anesthetic is required in this area to obtain profound anesthesia, if injected midway between the mesiobuccal and distobuccal roots.

- Palatal infiltration adjacent to the apex of the palatal root in maxillary molars is usually sufficient to obtain profound anesthesia required for root canal treatment

---

* * * * *   Clinical Note   * * * * *

Palatal anesthesia is often a very painful injection, even when performed by the most experienced clinician. However, temporary anesthesia before injection can be achieved in the following manner. Immediately before injection, place the opposite end of a mirror handle on the area to be anesthetized and apply firm pressure on palatal tissues (causing blanching of the soft tissue). Slowly slide the mirror handle 2-3 mm from the area of blanching and immediately penetrate the tissue with the needle. Maintain pressure on the mirror handle and inject the anesthetic slowly. This often eliminates the severe pain experienced during palatal injections. The technique will work for both infiltration and block anesthesia on the palate.

- A size 30 g needle is adequate for all palatal infiltration and block techniques

- Some controversy exists regarding the ability for a 30 g needle to aspirate blood in the same manner as a 25 g or 27 g

Mandibular Anterior and Premolar Teeth

- An inferior alveolar nerve block is required to obtain profound anesthesia for all mandibular anterior teeth
- Infiltration techniques are contraindicated for root canal therapy in anterior teeth
- Additional infiltration is not required routinely after an inferior alveolar nerve block during root canal therapy as both lingual and buccal soft tissues are adequately anesthetized with this technique
- Unless the patient demonstrates both lingual and buccal anesthesia, do not begin root canal therapy

---

* * * * * Clinical Note * * * * *

Although a mental nerve block can provide adequate anesthesia for root canal therapy in anterior and premolar teeth, the alveolar nerve block is preferred and more predictable in most cases. Lingual anesthesia must still be provided in premolars and, therefore, there is minimal advantage to this technique.

- Infiltration techniques will not provide profound anesthesia in mandibular premolars

Mandibular Molar Teeth

- Inferior alveolar nerve block and long buccal nerve infiltration is sufficient in most cases to provide profound anesthesia for root canal therapy in all mandibular molar teeth
- Buccal infiltration assures adequate anesthesia of the long buccal nerve for mesiobuccal and distobuccal roots of molars
- Lingual anesthesia (usually achieved with the inferior alveolar nerve block) is essential when performing root canal treatment in mandibular molars
- Lingual nerve innervation occurs in the mesiolingual and distolingual roots of mandibular molars
- Complete anesthesia of the lip (lip signs) should be achieved before proceeding with any root canal treatment
- To determine proper lip signs, an explorer tip should be gently depressed into the lip without discomfort to the patient

> * * * * * **Clinical Note** * * * * *
>
> At the onset of both lip signs and lingual nerve anesthesia the
> rubber dam can be placed. It is prudent to wait several
> minutes before beginning root canal treatment on a
> "hot tooth" as premature entry into the pulp
> chamber will cause increased discom-
> fort and a seemingly lowered
> pain threshold.

- In most cases, only one carpule of anesthetic is necessary for profound anesthesia in mandibular molars

- The needle tip should be placed completely through the soft tissue and gently pressed upon the ramus in order to achieve proper anesthesia

- The anesthetic solution should be injected very slowing immediately upon penetrating the oral soft tissues thus providing minimal discomfort to the patient

- 30 g short needles are contraindicated when attempting to achieve an inferior alveolar nerve block

- The use of a 25 g or 27 g long needle will provide adequate length and proper aspirating ability

> * * * * * **Clinical Note** * * * * *
>
> It is imperative when giving anesthesia, particularly block-type
> techniques, to aspirate multiple times during the injection of
> the anesthetic. During the course of an injection, the needle
> can move several millimeters once positioned along the
> ramus and can easily penetrate vessels unbeknownst
> to the clinician. The number of aspirations should
> be between 4 and 10 depending upon the
> speed at which the anesthesia is injected
> and the movement of the patient.

- Some clinicians recommend removing the needle and discarding the carpule if a positive aspiration of blood occurs during an injection

  - There is no scientific evidence that this provides any thera-peutic advantage to anesthesia than simply repositioning the needle tip and continuing with the injection

127

F. ADDITIONAL TECHNIQUES FOR OBTAINING ANESTHESIA

Gow-Gates Injection

- Described by Dr G Gow-Gates in 1973

- Will provide anesthesia of all components of the mandibular nerve

- Accurate administration of Gow-Gates will not require additional infiltration of other sites

- Technique requires insertion of needle to be both superior and more lateral with respect to the ramus

- Entire length of needle is usually almost completely buried within the soft tissue

- Multiple aspirations are essential to avoid injection into vessels, although vessels are not as dominant in the area of injection as in other types of nerve blocks

- Performed usually when routine inferior alveolar nerve block is inefficient in obtaining profound anesthesia

Periodontal Ligament Injection

- Used as an adjunct to infiltration and block techniques

- Will not usually provide profound anesthesia for root canal treatment in and of itself

- Injection occurs directly into the periodontal ligament usually on the mesial and distal surfaces of the desired tooth

- The term periodontal ligament injection is a misnomer as it is more appropriately named an intraosseous injection

- Only several drops of anesthetic will be deposited into the soft tissue during the injection

- Blanching of the soft tissue and significant resistance during injection assures proper technique

- Only short needles (25 g, 27 g, or 30 g) should be used for greater control during the procedure

- Technique suggests that the bevel of the needle be directed toward the bone; however, the clinical value of this is highly questionable

> ***** **Clinical Note** *****
>
> The anesthetic deposited with this technique does not limit
> itself solely to the injected tooth. The anesthesia will
> diffuse rapidly to adjacent teeth; however, adjacent
> teeth are usually not significantly anesthetized
> by this technique.

Intrapulpal Injection

- Reserved for "hot teeth" when all other techniques have failed to provide profound anesthesia

- Generally the most painful anesthetic technique

- Requires very little anesthetic solution of any type

- Small round bur (#2 or #4) is used to penetrate center of pulp chamber in short incremental "bursts"

> ***** **Clinical Note** *****
>
> When initial penetration of the pulp chamber with the bur is
> achieved, a 30 g needle is inserted into the access and
> with as much pressure as can be applied, the anesthetic
> is forced into the pulp chamber. At the same time the
> anesthetic solution is being deposited, the needle is
> advanced as deeply into the chamber as possible.
> If the needle can be forced into a canal, anes-
> thetic should be deposited into the canal
> also with the same procedure.

FREQUENTLY ASKED QUESTIONS (FAQs)

1. *I have a patient with a hot tooth. What's the best way to achieve anesthesia?*

   The best method to obtain profound anesthesia for a patient with a hot tooth is to use multiple injection techniques. After infiltration or block anesthesia, an intraligament injection is imperative. If this does not achieve your goal, a true intraosseous is another good choice. The most proven method, although also usually the most painful, is the intrapulpal.

2. *What the best anesthetic to use for root canal treatment in most patients?*

   There seems to be no agreement as to which is the "best" type. Xylocaine 2% with 1:100,000 epi is probably the best choice in most cases. Longer acting anesthetics or multiple injections do not necessarily provide a more profound anesthesia if the appropriate technique has been used.

3. **Should I use a topical anesthetic before injecting the patient?**

It depends. These work even if it is only a psychological result. However, a rapid shaking of the patient's oral soft tissues will also cause the same effect, take less time, and is less expensive.

Chapter XI

Treatment of Endodontic Emergencies

TREATMENT OF ENDODONTIC EMERGENCIES

A. DIAGNOSIS

- The most important factor in treating the endodontic emergency patient in moderate to severe pain is to obtain an expedient and accurate diagnosis

- The most appropriate treatment procedure is based on the diagnostic categories; therefore, it is imperative to arrive at the most logical diagnosis based on the clinical observations made by the clinician and the statements from the patient's chief complaint

- One of the most difficult decisions a clinician is faced with has to deal with treating the patient when there is uncertainty regarding the etiology of pain

- The astute clinician will not listen solely to the patient's complaints and, in some cases, the patient's diagnosis of which tooth is causing the problem

- The diagnosis must be a combination of the patient's description of the problem and the objective signs that the clinician can demonstrate

```
* * * * *   Clinical Note   * * * * *

No tooth should ever be endodontically treated unless the
     clinician is 90% or better assured that the correct
         diagnosis and correct tooth have been identified.
     This can often mean that a patient will be sent
         home without any endodontic treatment.
         The patient must be made to understand
             that the pain will localize and treat-
                 ment will be initiated at that point,
                     and only at that point in time.
```

B. REVERSIBLE PULPITIS

- Because the pulp is "reversibly" inflamed, the majority of reversible pulpitis cases require either the removal of the etiology or the "tincture of time"

- Removal of the causative agent may be the removal of incipient caries, covering exposed cervical dentin, smoothing and covering a fractured cusp, or the removal of fractured tooth structure

- Most reversible pulpitis cases are the result of basic restorative procedures that cause transient inflammation within the pulpal tissues

- Occasionally, continued mild pulpal pain from a seemingly benign procedure (Class I amalgam or simple composite restoration) will linger for several weeks

- If the pain lasts more than a week or two, occasionally the removal of the restoration and the placement of a sedative dressing will be helpful in alleviating the pain

---

***** Clinical Note *****

Whenever any tooth structure is removed or is affected by the procedure of removing a restoration for the purposes of placing a sedative dressing, there is always a probability that this procedure in and of itself will cause a reversible state to become irreversible in nature. Patients should always be cautioned that any restorative procedure has the potential to exacerbate symptoms already present from previous trauma.

C. IRREVERSIBLE PULPITIS (IP) WITH LOCALIZED PAIN

***** Clinical Note *****

All endodontic therapy (regardless of the diagnosis) must be performed under a rubber dam with the offending tooth properly isolated from salivary leakage.

IP-Anterior Teeth

- Once a definitive diagnosis of IP has been made, proper and expedient emergency treatment is required to prevent additional postoperative sequelae

- A pulpotomy procedure will resolve the patient's symptoms in most cases

- However, because in anterior teeth with IP, a pulpectomy procedure takes little additional time compared to a pulpotomy, the most appropriate treatment of choice is pulpectomy

***** **Clinical Note** *****

If the patient is percussion-sensitive, it is imperative that a pulpectomy be performed. Otherwise, there is a high probability that mastication sensitivity will not be relieved.

- Every attempt should be made to remove the pulpal tissue in a complete manner versus lacerating the soft tissue and, thereby, inducing a high potential for additional hemorrhage

- The most ideal method for removing vital and nonvital pulpal tissue is accomplished by using the largest hedström file that will fit into the canal to the estimated WL

  - The file is twisted into the soft tissue as far into the canal as possible and the tissue removed as it becomes twisted upon the file

  - Every attempt should be made to prevent lacerating and causing additional damage to the vital tissue as this may result in additional pain and postoperative symptoms

***** **Clinical Note** *****

There is some controversy regarding whether reduction of the occlusion will actually reduce the postoperative pain of the patient. However, because there are no negative sequelae to adjusting the occlusion, it is best to perform this procedure whenever there is reported pain or tenderness reported to mastication or frank percussion sensitivity noted by the clinician.

IP-Posterior Teeth (Multirooted)

- If no mastication sensitivity is reported, a pulpotomy is often sufficient in most cases to reduce the patient's symptoms

- In patients reporting mastication sensitivity or if there is frank percussion sensitivity, a pulpectomy should be performed on all roots, if possible

  - In cases where time is limited, a pulpotomy with the additional procedure of a pulpectomy on the largest root (maxillary palatal roots and mandibular distal roots) is the treatment of choice

  - In these situations, the largest file that will bind only to the soft tissue and not to the walls of the dentin should be inserted into the largest canal and a "one-step" pulpectomy should be performed

- Large single rooted premolars (both maxillary and mandibular) can be treated in a similar fashion as anterior teeth with respect to pulpectomy procedures

---

* * * * * Clinical Note * * * * *

All canals should be instrumented to at least a size 25 K file in order to achieve appropriate debridement of the canals.

D. IRREVERSIBLE PULPITIS WITH NONLOCALIZED PAIN

- The patient has been in moderate to severe pain and may present to the office in acute pain; however, no diagnostic tests will confirm or negate a specific tooth

  - Often one or more teeth may be sensitive to percussion, but one tooth does not cause significantly more pain than the others in the area where the patient is complaining of discomfort

  - Cold and heat tests are all within normal limits as is palpation and all additional tests

- Radiographic evidence is the only definitive method for determining which tooth is the etiology of pain

  - On occasion, the clinician may determine that the periodontal ligament space is widened or the lamina dura has thickened significantly in addition to the widened periodontal ligament space

  - However, radiographs are often within normal limits, especially in the early stages of IP or in posterior mandibular teeth with dense cortical plates

---

* * * * * Clinical Note * * * * *

The clinician must be careful when assessing radiographs for periapical changes especially when under the perceived pressure to make a diagnosis because of a patient's discomfort level. Historical films of the tooth (teeth) in question must be examined carefully and compared to current films. When the radiographs are unremarkable and clinical signs/symptoms provide no additional diagnostic support, a wait-and-watch response by the clinician is the most appropriate treatment for the patient.

- In most cases of irreversible pulpitis with nonlocalized symptoms, the patient should be sent home with appropriate analgesics (if necessary) and instructed to return when the pain localizes

---

***** **Clinical Note** *****

Antibiotics are rarely (if ever) indicated for patients with non-localized irreversible pulpitis. There are three main indications for the use of antibiotics when dealing with lesions of endodontic origin (irreversible pulpitis and necrotic pulps). Antibiotics are indicated in the patient who presents with lymphadenopathy, cellulitis, and/or a fever greater>100°F.

- The histopathology of disease dictates that the symptoms will localize to a specific tooth whereby the clinician will be able to diagnose accurately and to treat appropriately

E. NECROTIC PULP – NO SWELLING – NO SINUS TRACT

NP-Anterior Teeth

- With necrotic pulps in anterior teeth, the tissue must be removed completely from the canal system in order to alleviate the symptoms.

- Two approaches can be utilized to accomplish this objective

  - Often, a pulpectomy procedure can be utilized to remove the tissue within the canal system using the largest hedström file that will fit to the estimated WL without impinging on the hard tissues

    - The file is twisted in a clockwise manner into the soft tissue until the estimated WL is achieved

    - The file is then removed with the necrotic pulp tissue twisted around the file

    - There is no need for significant additional instrumentation of the hard and soft tissue of the canal; however, copious amounts of sodium hypochlorite (50% dilution) are utilized in the debridement process and after the tissue has been removed

      - This technique prevents inadvertent debris from being pushed out the apex and causing additional discomfort

- After removal of the soft tissue, the hedström file should be used in a flaring motion against the sides of the canal to remove the remaining soft tissue with the canal being completely filled with sodium hypochlorite

---

***** **Clinical Note** *****

Complete debridement of the necrotic tissue within the canal system must be accomplished in order to eliminate patient symptoms. If tissue is left behind, bacteria can again proliferate and cause additional symptoms.

NP-Posterior Teeth

- Pulpotomy is contraindicated as an emergency procedure in necrotic posterior teeth

- Two treatment regimes are suggested because of the high likelihood that the smaller roots (mesial roots of mandibular molars and buccal roots of maxillary molars) have one or more calcified canals

- **METHOD I**

  - Estimate WL of all canals from start film or use an apex locator and debride the coronal 2/3 of all canals beginning with a size 10-15 K file and work up to a size 25 K file in all canals

  - Copious amounts of sodium hypochlorite (50% dilution) should be used throughout the procedure

  - In method I, the clinician must be careful to prevent ledging and/or blockage of the remaining apical 1/3 of the canal

    - To prevent blockage or ledging, a 10-15 K file should be placed into the canal to the estimated WL after each file has been used for cleaning

  - With an air syringe, carefully dry the pulp chamber, place a sterile cotton pellet in the chamber, and close with temporary

---

***** **Clinical Note** *****

The use of any of the popular intracanal medicaments (Formocresol, CMCP, Cresatin, etc) is unwarranted and provides no additional therapeutic advantage. Therefore, a sterile cotton pellet is all that is necessary.

- **METHOD II (Preferred Method)**

  - Determine correct WL in all canals

  - Completely instrument all canals to a size 25 K file using copious amounts of sodium hypochlorite

  - With an air syringe, carefully dry the pulp chamber, place a sterile cotton pellet in the chamber and close with temporary

---

***** Clinical Note *****

It is not necessary to completely dry the canals with paper points. The sodium hypochlorite that remains will maintain an aseptic environment within the canal system without causing any periapical symptoms.

F. NECROTIC PULP – NO SWELLING – SINUS TRACT PRESENT

***** Clinical Note *****

One appointment endodontics is contraindicated in few cases. However, with respect to symptoms and one appointment root canal therapy, the presence of a patent sinus tract will provide the highest probability that no post-operative symptoms will result after instrumentation and obturation of the root canal system in one appointment.

- It is very unusual for a patient to be in any pain with a draining sinus tract present

- Most patients with draining sinus tracts are asymptomatic or have had an episode of moderate to severe pain until the sinus became patent

- All sinus tracts should be traced to their etiology

  - Sinus tracts are best traced with a minimum of a size #30 gutta-percha cone

  - When inserting the gutta-percha cone into the sinus tract, it is advisable to proceed slowly and let the gutta-percha cone warm as it is inserted

- This will cause less pain to the patient as the warmed
  GP point will more easily flex and bend to accommodate the soft tissue structure of the tract

- All tracings should be radiographed to determine the
  etiology of the sinus tract

- Sinus tracings can determine whether the etiology of the
  swelling and discomfort is periodontal and/or endodontic in
  nature

- **ANTERIOR TEETH**

  - WL, complete debridement, and obturation of the root
    canal system

- **POSTERIOR TEETH**

  - **Method II** (under **NP-Posterior Teeth**) is preferred;
    however, if time allows, complete instrumentation and
    obturation of the root canal system is justified

G. NECROTIC PULP – LOCALIZED INTRAORAL SWELLING PRESENT

***** Clinical Note *****

Localized intraoral swelling is not an indication for antibiotics.
By removing the etiology (necrotic pulpal tissue) the
swelling will resolve without the need for
pharmacotherapeutics.

- With intraoral swelling, the clinician must remove as much of
  the etiology (necrotic pulpal tissue) as possible

- Treatment — **Method II** (under **NP-Posterior Teeth**) is
  preferred

***** Clinical Note *****

The patient should be made aware that after instrumentation
of a necrotic tooth in the presence (or absence) of localized
intraoral swelling that some additional swelling and/or pain
is not uncommon and should be expected
for a couple of days.

- If the tissue is fluctuant (semi-solid mass which moves or
  depresses upon palpation), an incision and drainage procedure

can be performed; however, it is not always indicated depending upon the size of the swelling

- **Tissue fluctuant and drainage obtained through tooth**
    - Access opening, establish drainage, biomechanical instrumentation of tooth (Method I or II), cotton pellet and temporary
    - Perform incision and drainage, if indicated
        - Obtain adequate anesthesia by injecting <u>around and not into</u> the fluctuant area
        - Incision with #12 or #15 scalpel blade to bone
        - Hemostats are then used in an opening and closing method to disrupt areas of loculated purulence
        - Drains are not indicated as the incision usually remains open an adequate amount of time to allow discharge of all materials
    - Prescribe warm saline rinses

- **Tissue fluctuant but no drainage obtained through tooth**
    - Access opening, no drainage obtained, biomechanical instrumentation of tooth (Method I or II), cotton pellet and temporary
    - Perform incision and drainage if indicated
    - Prescribe warm saline rinses

- **Tissue nonfluctuant and drainage through the tooth**
    - Access opening, establish drainage through tooth, biomechanical instrumentation of tooth (Method I or II), cotton pellet and temporary
    - Incision and drainage not indicated
    - Antibiotics indicated only if a cellulitis is present in addition to the localized swelling

- **Tissue nonfluctuant and no drainage through the tooth**
    - Access opening, no drainage established through tooth, biomechanical instrumentation of tooth (Method I or II), cotton pellet and temporary
    - Incision and drainage not indicated
    - Prescribe warm saline rinses
    - Antibiotics indicated if cellulitis and/or fever and/or lymphadenopathy

H. NECROTIC PULP – EXTRAORAL SWELLING PRESENT (CELLULITIS)

- Antibiotics are indicated in cases of cellulitis

  - Loading dose of 1-2 g of Pen VK then 500 mg every 6 hours for 7-10 days

  - Cephalosporins are alternative choice if patient is allergic to penicillin

---

* * * * *   Clinical Note   * * * * *

There is a reported 20% cross reactivity (allergic reaction) in patients with a definitive history of immediate reaction to penicillin.

  - Erythromycins are next alternative followed by clindamycin and metronidazole

- In cases of cellulitis, it is imperative to remove the etiology as quickly as possible; therefore, opening the tooth and biomechanical instrumentation is indicated at the emergency appointment, if at all possible

- Complete debridement of the canal system should take place at the emergency visit

---

* * * * *   Clinical Note   * * * * *

Although one appointment endodontics is not contraindicated in a patient with a cellulitis, the majority of clinicians are more comfortable in performing only the emergency procedure at this visit. The patient should return for follow-up within 2-5 days after the emergency appointment at which time the endodontic procedure can be completed, if desired.

- Treatment — **Method II** (under **NP-Posterior Teeth**) is preferred (see treatment of NP-Localized Tissue Swelling-Tissue Nonfluctuant)

***** Clinical Note *****

In endodontic infections, antibiotics do not usually demonstrate
their effectiveness within the first 24-48 hours. The clinician
must realize this and determine if the patient's signs and
symptoms are exacerbating or simply maintaining a
status quo. Switching antibiotics before a minimum
of 2-3 days is contraindicated unless the fever
and/or swelling are becoming significantly
worsened. If the swelling and the temperature
of the patient remains about the same as
that of the emergency visit, then there
is a high likelihood that the antibiotics
are performing appropriately.

I. OBTAINING ADEQUATE ANESTHESIA

- Patients with highly inflamed cases of irreversible pulpitis are
  often difficult to anesthetize with conventional techniques

    - Block anesthesia is indicated always before adjunctive
      methods are employed

    - If adequate anesthesia cannot be obtained conventionally,
      a periodontal ligament injection is employed

    - When PDL injections are inadequate, an intrapulpal has an
      extremely high degree of success if performed appropri-
      ately

        - Because the patient is usually sensitive to cold liquids
          and/or air, the water should be turned off of the high
          speed handpiece

        - A #1/2 or #2 round bur should be used to penetrate
          the pulp chamber

        - A #30 or #27 short needle is positioned into the pulp
          chamber and anesthetic injected

***** Clinical Note *****

It is not the injected anesthetic into the pulpal tissue which
causes profound anesthesia but rather the pressure of
the liquid. Therefore, it is not significant to select
a specific anesthetic, as saline would also
cause pulpal anesthesia in these cases.

J. ANALGESICS FOR POSTOPERATIVE PAIN AFTER EMERGENCY TREATMENT

- Most dental pain is a result of inflammation
    - The analgesics of choice for pain of endodontic origin are the nonsteroidal anti-inflammatory agents
        - Ibuprofen — 600-800 mg doses usually sufficient for most dental pain
        - Other examples: Fenoprofen, flurbiprofen, and naproxen
    - When narcotic agents are required, the drugs of choice are Tylenol® #3, Vicodan®, Vicodan® ES, and Percodan®

***** Clinical Note *****

The vast majority of patients will respond favorably with proper endodontic treatment and over-the-counter nonsteroidal anti-inflammatory agents. The clinician should be aware of the high potential for drug abuse and the extremely common excuse that the endodontic therapy is not working properly, thereby necessitating pre- scriptions for narcotic agents. It is rare that a patient does not respond favorably within 24-48 hours after appropriate endodontic therapy.

FREQUENTLY ASKED QUESTIONS (FAQs)

1. *Why does my tooth hurt after the nerve has been removed?*

    After root canal therapy, particularly in emergency treatment situations, the tenderness and pain associated postopera- tively is not from the tooth itself. Rather, the surrounding bone and/or periodontal ligament are both potentially inflamed. Because the same "nerve" which innervates the tooth also innervates the surrounding tissues, the pain is perceived from the tooth rather than the actual source, the PDL and periradicular tissues.

2. *The pain stopped when I got this gum boil. It doesn't hurt anymore, why do I still need the root canal?*

    The pain was relieved because of the drainage obtained when the gum boil burst. However, there is still an infection in this tooth which will not go away until the tooth is either extracted or has root canal treatment to remove the dead tissue and the bacteria which is inside the tooth. In addition, if the gum boil closes over, there may be additional pain which will return.

3. *I usually stop taking the antibiotics when the pain and swelling goes away — why should I continue with the drug for the full 7 days?*

Patients who do not take their antibiotics for the full course as prescribed run the risk of developing bacteria which are no longer sensitive or are immune to the antibiotic. In patients in whom this occurs, the next time this medication is prescribed, there is a significant decrease in the ability for the drug to perform its antibiotic action. The bacteria can, therefore, continue growing and cause serious symptoms and problems for the patient.

Chapter XII

Treatment of
Traumatic Injuries

TREATMENT OF TRAUMATIC INJURIES

A. AVULSION INJURIES

Guidelines for Treating the Avulsed Tooth

- There are several sets of guidelines available regarding the appropriate treatment for a patient with an avulsed tooth

  - American Association of Endodontists, October 1995

  - Andreasen and Andreasen, *Textbook and Color Atlas of Traumatic Injuries to Teeth*, 1994

  - "Protocols for Clinical Pediatric Dentistry," *The Journal of Pedodontics*, 3rd ed, 1995, 31-2

  - Roberts and Longhurst, *Oral and Dental Trauma in Children and Adolescents*, 1st ed, 1996

---

* * * * *   Clinical Note   * * * * *

Although many of the guidelines for treatment of the avulsed tooth are based on sound research and clinical studies, there is a great need for additional research support for the basis of some of the suggested treatment modalities. The guidelines suggested in this chapter are a combination of both authors' experience and research in this area as well as the suggestions from the published guidelines.

Emergency Treatment at the Site of Trauma

- Rinse tooth with sterile saline, milk, or water and replant into socket as soon as possible

- If possible, do not scrape or damage the root

- Have patient bite gently on gauze or cloth or have patient secure tooth in socket with finger pressure

- Patient should see dentist or hospital-based emergency dental clinic immediately

- If patient or individual at injury site cannot perform replantation, tooth should be placed into a liquid medium immediately

  - Milk, Hank's balanced salt solution (HBSS), 3M™ Save-A-Tooth™ System, saline, secure tooth in plastic wrap, or place into patient's mouth or water as the two least desirable choices

```
* * * * *   Clinical Note   * * * * *
```
Tooth must be kept hydrated and should not be exposed to an
environment that will allow the cells to necrose. By maintaining the cellular integrity of the root surface,
a better prognosis will result.

Emergency Treatment in Dental Office – Tooth Already Replanted in Socket

- Assure that the tooth was replanted correctly and is clinically in normal alignment with other teeth and adjacent arch

- Expose a radiograph to verify the avulsed tooth (teeth) is/are in correct alignment, there are no foreign objects within the socket, and there are no alveolar fractures present

    - In the presence of alveolar fractures, a longer splinting period is warranted, usually a minimum of 6-8 weeks

    - A more rigid splint is also indicated when alveolar fractures are present

- Splint avulsed tooth in normal anatomical position with composite alone, composite with wire, or orthodontic brackets, wire, and composite

```
* * * * *   Clinical Note   * * * * *
```
Any accepted splinting method that will function to hold the
traumatized tooth in place is appropriate. The clinician
should have no concern regarding the use of a rigid
versus "physiologic" splint. Research supports
either method will stabilize the tooth
without negative sequelae.

- Splint should remain in place for 7-14 days or longer if avulsed tooth is too mobile for splint to be removed

```
* * * * *   Clinical Note   * * * * *
```
Most avulsed teeth in the absence of other complications will
be firm within 5-7 days. It is uncommon for an avulsed
tooth to require splinting beyond 2 weeks.

- Tetanus booster or immunization should be considered with any avulsion injury

Closed Apex

- If the tooth has a closed apex, patient should be informed that a root canal procedure is required

  - Revascularization of closed apex teeth is extremely remote and, therefore, is not usually a consideration

  - Root canal therapy may be initiated at the time of splinting or should be initiated within 2 weeks of the injury for the best prognosis

---

***** **Clinical Note** *****

One of the most serious problems associated with avulsed teeth is that of inflammatory root resorption. This process is very destructive and the extremely rapid resorption can usually be controlled by timely and appropriate root canal treatment of the avulsed tooth.

Open Apex

- If the tooth has an open apex, consider the potential for revascularization of the pulp in lieu of endodontic therapy

- The avulsed tooth must be closely monitored, usually on a weekly basis for the first 8 weeks

- Radiographic evidence of revascularization and the lack of periradicular pathosis must be confirmed

- Periapical radiographs should be taken at least every other week for the first 8 weeks in order to compare the avulsed tooth's apical anatomy with the contralateral tooth

- Should definitive evidence of periradicular pathosis (radiolucent areas of resorption of cementum/dentin/bone) be noted, root canal therapy must be instituted immediately

---

***** **Clinical Note** *****

The patient should be made aware of the critical necessity for follow-up care. Inflammatory root resorption is an asymptomatic process and the patient will likely be completely unaware of its destructive nature. If it occurs in a young patient with a large open apex, the root of the avulsed tooth could be completely resorbed in as little as 2-3 months without appropriate intervention by the clinician.

Recommended Guidelines of the American Association of Endodontists, October 1995*

Open Apex and <60 Minutes Extraoral Dry Time*

- Replant tooth with the intent of achieving revascularization
- Recall patient every 3-4 weeks
- If evidence of periapical pathosis is noted, the canal(s) should be instrumented and treated with calcium hydroxide in an attempt to achieve apexification

Open Apex and >60 Minutes Extraoral Dry Time*

- Instrument canal(s) and obturate with calcium hydroxide
- Place patient on 6- to 8-week recall
- Other options should be presented to the patient because of poor prognosis

Partially to Completely Closed Apex and <60 Minutes Extraoral Dry Time*

- Instrument canal(s) within 7-14 days
- Place calcium hydroxide in the canal(s) for as long as practical (6-12 months)
- Permanently obturate with gutta-percha and sealer

Partially to Completely Closed Apex and >60 Minutes Extraoral Dry Time*

- Instrument canal(s) intraorally or extraorally
- Before replanting tooth into alveolar socket, remove tissue tags from root and soak tooth in an accepted dental fluoride solution

---

* * * * *   Clinical Note   * * * * *

There are numerous studies which support replanting a tooth regardless of the amount of time in which it was extraoral. Some studies have indicated that up to 45 days is still within reasonable limits. Therefore, teeth which have been extraoral and either stored in a liquid medium or stored dry should be replanted, regardless of their time out of the socket.

Prognosis of Avulsed Teeth

- The prognosis of an avulsed tooth is dependent upon multiple factors such as extraoral dry time, apex development (age of patient), damage to the root surface, and timely and appropriate treatment

- All patients with an avulsed tooth should be told that the prognosis is "guarded" at best because, even under "ideal" conditions, an avulsed tooth may undergo rapid (inflammatory) or slow (replacement) resorption resulting in the loss of the tooth

---

***** **Clinical Note** *****

On the average, older patients have a better prognosis with avulsion injuries than younger patients. This is a result of multiple factors including the pulp chamber and root canal system usually being smaller and the dentinal tubules being more sclerotic resulting in less communication between the root canal system and the cementum and periodontal tissues.

B. LUXATION INJURIES

- There are five types of luxation injuries treated according their classification

- The overall prognosis of luxation injuries is excellent to very good depending upon their classification

- All patients who experience a luxation injury should be informed that the pulpal prognosis is usually very good; there is always the possibility that a root canal will be necessary at some time in the future

C. CLASSIFICATION OF LUXATION INJURIES

In order of severity:

1. Concussion
2. Subluxation
3. Extrusive luxation
4. Lateral luxation
5. Intrusive luxation

***** **Clinical Note** *****

When splinting is indicated in any luxation or avulsion injury, a
physiological, semirigid, or rigid splint is acceptable. Bonding
to adjacent teeth with composite or using an orthodontic
bracket and wire is also suitable. one tooth on either
side of the traumatized tooth should be
included in the splint.

---

1. **CONCUSSION INJURY**

   – A relatively minor injury to the tooth resulting in percussion
     sensitivity but without mobility

   – No splinting is required since mobility is usually within
     normal limits

   – Palliative treatment only, usually consisting of reduction of
     the occlusal forces on the tooth

   – Patient should be recalled within 1-2 weeks

   – Root canal therapy is not indicated in the majority of
     concussion injuries

   – Within 1-2 weeks, the traumatized tooth should be WNL to
     all clinical tests including percussion, palpation, and vitality
     tests

   – In the absence of radiographic changes, root canal therapy
     is not indicated

2. **SUBLUXATION INJURY**

   – More severe than concussion injuries

   – Splinting is not required usually, although the mobility is
     similar to a periodontally involved tooth (+1 to +2 mm) and
     splinting can be performed if considered necessary

   – Palliative treatment only, usually consisting of reduction of
     the occlusal forces on the tooth

   – Patient should be recalled within 1-2 weeks

   – Root canal therapy is indicated in <20% of the cases of
     subluxation injuries

   – Long-term sequelae, although not highly probable, include
     calcification of the pulp chamber and/or canal system or
     necrosis of the pulp, marginal bone loss

   – External and/or internal resorption does not generally
     occur

3. **EXTRUSIVE LUXATION INJURY**

   – More severe than subluxation

   – Administer local anesthetic and reposition tooth in socket

   – Splinting is generally required for 7-14 days

   – Root canal therapy required in majority of cases

   – Patient should be recalled within 1-2 weeks

***** **Clinical Note** *****

EPT and thermal tests may not provide accurate data within
the first several weeks post-trauma. To determine vitality
status of pulp in the absence of radiographic signs
or symptoms, patient should be recalled in
6-8 weeks and vitality tests should be
performed at that time.

   – Long-term sequelae include high probability of pulpal
     necrosis and marginal bone loss is possible

   – External and/or internal resorption is not likely; however, a
     greater probability of external resorption will result if
     severe damage occurs to the PDL

4. **LATERAL LUXATION INJURY**

   – More severe than extrusive since damage to the bone
     often occurs

   – Administer local anesthetic and reposition tooth in socket

   – Splinting is required for 7-14 days or longer (2-8 weeks) if
     bony fractures are noted

   – Root canal therapy indicated in majority of cases

   – Long-term sequelae include high probability of pulpal
     necrosis and marginal bone loss is possible

   – External and/or internal resorption is unlikely

5. **INTRUSIVE LUXATION INJURY**

   – Most severe of all luxation injuries

   – Patient should be told that prognosis is guarded

- Optimal treatment has not been established; therefore, select one of the following three methods

  Option I: Allow tooth to erupt on its own

  - This should occur within the first 2-4 weeks after injury

  - If tooth does not spontaneously erupt within 2-4 weeks, attempt Option II

  - Younger patients have higher probability for spontaneous eruption than older patients

  Option II: Place orthodontic wire on tooth and extrude

  - Extrusion should occur over several weeks

  Option III: Use forceps to extract tooth into normal position

  - Tooth should be splinted immediately after repositioning

- Root canal therapy is indicated in all closed apex cases

  - Open apex cases should be monitored extremely closely as external resorption may play a major role in tooth loss

- External root resorption (replacement resorption) is highly probable and will likely lead to the loss of the tooth

  - Replacement resorption is chronic in nature and, therefore, very slow; tooth loss will usually take many years with this type of resorption

D. TYPICAL SEQUELAE OF LUXATION INJURIES

Pulp Canal Obliteration

- Usually <40% of the cases of all luxation injuries undergo pulp canal obliteration

---

***** **Clinical Note** *****

Although the pulp chamber and root canal system may undergo calcification changes, this is not an indication to initiate root canal therapy. Most teeth that become calcified as a result of trauma, etc, do not become necrotic after the calcification process commences.

Marginal Bone Loss

- Usually <25% of the teeth with luxation injures have marginal bone loss

- The amount of bone loss is generally minor when it does occur

Transient Apical Breakdown

- A radiolucency persists over an extended period of time (up to 12 months)

- Usually <5% probability of it occurring

- No treatment required as it will resolve spontaneously

Discoloration of the Crown

- Depending upon the color, assess if treatment is indicated

    - When coronal color change is yellow in hue and there is no radiographic evidence of a pulp chamber, probability exists that because of the pulp chamber obliteration with dentin, the color change has resulted and no treatment is required regardless of the EPT/thermal test results

    - If coronal color change is dark gray to brown, there is a higher likelihood that the pulp contents have broken down and have diffused into the dentinal tubules. Root canal therapy is generally indicated after vitality tests and/or radiographic evidence supports treatment.

E. HORIZONTAL ROOT FRACTURES

- A fracture of the root of a tooth that involves cementum, dentin, and root canal system

    Classification:

    1. Apical Third Fracture
    2. Middle Third Fracture
    3. Coronal Third Fracture

    1. **APICAL THIRD FRACTURES**

        - Expose radiograph before tooth is repositioned in order to determine extent of fracture

        - Reposition coronal segment if displaced and expose additional radiograph to assure complete reapproximation

- Splinting is indicated if coronal segment is mobile (6-8 weeks – rigid splint); however, because most horizontal root fractures occur in anterior maxillary teeth, the roots are sufficiently long which stabilizes the coronal segment

***** Clinical Note *****

Splint two teeth on either side of fractured tooth to assure rigidity of the splint. Use orthodontic wire and orthodontic brackets to assure rigidity and security of the splint. The splint must be secure for 6-8 weeks in order to assure proper healing of the fractured segments.

- Root canal therapy is not usually indicated unless symptoms, signs, or radiographic evidence indicate therapy is required
- Because this type of tooth trauma is severe, vitality tests should be performed at time of splint removal unless symptoms indicate pulpal pathosis

***** Clinical Note *****

If root canal therapy is indicated, only the coronal segment should be treated. The apical segment maintains its vitality in most cases of horizontal root fractures. In addition, the apical segment will usually calcify.

2. MIDDLE THIRD FRACTURES

- Expose radiograph before tooth is repositioned in order to determine extent of fracture
- Reposition coronal segment if displaced and expose additional radiograph to assure complete reapproximation
- Coronal segment will require splinting after repositioning is completed
- Splint with rigid splint for 6-8 weeks

***** Clinical Note *****

Pathognomonic for a failing union between the two segments is a semilunar radiolucency on one or both sides of the fracture line.

- If root canal therapy is indicated from radiographs, patient symptoms, or clinical tests, perform endodontics only in the coronal half of the root; the apical half will likely maintain its vitality

158

3. CORONAL THIRD FRACTURES

- Most difficult for clinician to treat

- Depending upon the location of the fracture, the tooth may be treated conservatively; however, most often the coronal segment is very mobile and difficult to immobilize

- Expose radiograph before tooth is repositioned in order to determine extent of fracture

- Reposition coronal segment if displaced and expose additional radiograph to assure complete reapproximation

---

***** **Clinical Note** *****

The clinician should always periodontally probe the coronal third of a horizontally root fractured tooth. If the fracture site can be probed, then the prognosis is very poor. Salivary contamination of the fracture site will likely prevent normal healing. In addition, it is extremely difficult to splint rigidly the coronal third to the apical two-thirds because of the damage that has occurred to both the tooth structure and to the alveolar bone.

- Splint with rigid splint for 6-8 weeks

- Warn patient about poor prognosis and likelihood that coronal tooth structure will be lost

- Depending upon the site of the fracture, the apical segment may be extruded into position if the coronal segment is lost

• HEALING OF HORIZONTAL ROOT FRACTURES

3 types of healing are possible:

1. Calcified union between segments (ideal type of healing)

    - This type of healing occurs when both segments are reapproximated correctly and the coronal segment was stable during the healing process

    - Radiographically, the fracture site is calcified and the two segments have a normal anatomy, although in some cases, a slight radiolucency within the fracture site can be noted

2. Soft tissue union between segments

   – A connective tissue union forms between the two segments

   – A radiolucency is present along the fracture site

3. Bone and connective tissue healing

   – Usually occurs in younger patients when maxilla is still in development stage

   – Radiographically, the two segments are separated by a segment of bone, each root having its own PDL

- **FAILURE OF TWO SEGMENTS TO HEAL**

  – Occurs when there is a failure of the two segments to calcify or to heal with a soft tissue union

  – Usually occurs because of the level of the fracture site being close to the epithelial attachment or improper stabilization of the two segments

  – A sinus tract may form or the ability to probe to the fracture site indicating salivary contamination of the fracture and inability to heal properly

  – A semilunar radiolucency is noted on one or both sides of the root fracture (pathognomonic for this type of failing union between the two segments)

  – Root canal therapy is indicated because the coronal segment is nonvital

  – Prognosis is poor to guarded

  – Additional stabilization is generally required

Chapter XIII

Resorption

RESORPTION

I. Root Resorption Nomenclature

A. INTERNAL ROOT RESORPTION (IRR)

Nonperforating IRR

- A defect that occurs within the pulp chamber and/or anywhere within the root canal system that causes destruction of the dentin

- Specific etiology for internal resorption is unknown

- The following have been implicated as predisposing factors for internal root resorption

    - Chronic inflammation within the pulp chamber/canal system

    - Bacteria may also play a significant role

    - Trauma

    - Caries

    - May be induced by restorative procedures

        - Large and/or deep restorations

        - Crown/bridge preparations

        - Any procedure that causes a moderate to severe amount of pulpal inflammation

    - Pulp capping procedures

    - Pulpotomy procedures

- Can occur with equal frequency in the apical, middle, or coronal 1/3 or the root

- Occurs with less frequency solely within the pulp chamber

- Occurs more frequently in older patients, but is not limited to adult patients

- Resorptive process rate can range from chronic (very slow) to extremely rapid

- The dentinal tubules have been implicated as one method for the rate and the architecture of destructive nature of internal resorption

```
* * * * *    Clinical Note    * * * * *
```

The prognosis is very good to excellent for nonperforating
internal resorption, if treated in a timely manner. Overall,
the prognosis is more a function of the involved
tooth's restorability since the endodontic
success rate is going to be the same as
that for other endodontically-treated
teeth (85% to 95%).

Perforating IRR

- An internal defect that occurs within the pulp chamber and/or anywhere within the root canal system that causes destruction of dentin and the cementum or enamel

- There is communication with the periodontium and/or the intra-oral environment

- Usually a more severe type of resorption because of the additional therapy required to resolve the defect

```
* * * * *    Clinical Note    * * * * *
```

It is imperative to treat expediently teeth that have been diagnosed with perforating internal root resorption. Treatment
should be initiated within several days to one week
after diagnosis of this condition. There is a high
likelihood that the resorption process will
destroy significant amounts of root
surface in as little as 6-12 weeks.

- Often has a poor to guarded prognosis depending upon the area where the external defect occurs

- Will require usually both nonsurgical and surgical procedures for a successful outcome

B. EXTERNAL ROOT RESORPTION (ERR)

Surface Root Resorption

- Initiated on the root surface of the tooth
- Resorption of the cementum and occasionally the dentin
- Usually a self-limiting process
- Can be a physiological and normal process of remodeling the surface of the root
- Cannot be detected routinely with bitewing or periapical films

- Usually small pockets of resorption are present and are limited in size and number on the root surface

- Usually evident upon histological examination only

- Probably occurs during conservative orthodontic therapy

Inflammatory Root Resorption

- Most severe type of resorption

- Initiated on the root surface of the tooth

- Osteoclastic/dentinoclastic cells destroy the cementum and dentin

- Scooped out areas of tooth structure is replaced by granulation tissue/inflammatory cells

- Extremely rapid process

- Extensive destruction (resorption) of the cementum and the dentin

- Not a self-limiting process

- **Requires immediate attention**

- Usually a result of several factors that provide an optimal environment in which it can occur

    - bacteria

    - damage to the periodontium

    - necrotic pulpal tissue

- Patients are generally asymptomatic and unaware of the severe nature of this type of resorption

---

* * * * * Clinical Note * * * * *

It is imperative to treat teeth that have been diagnosed with inflammatory root resorption as soon as possible. If treatment cannot be initiated within several days to one week after diagnosis of this condition, there is a high likelihood that the resorption process will destroy the entire root surface in as little as 6-12 weeks.

- Radiographically, this type of resorption is noted for its scooped out radiolucent areas of tooth structure

- Can occur along any surface of the root where damage to the periodontium has occurred

- Usually large areas of the tooth are affected and there is no limit to the number of areas or to the size of damage

- Occurs primarily in teeth after avulsion injuries and to some extent after certain types of luxation injuries, primarily intrusive luxation

Replacement Root Resorption

- A chronic type of process that usually occurs over several months to years
- Resorption is initiated on the root surface of the tooth
- Although any tooth may be affected by external replacement resorption, it is most often seen as a sequelae to avulsion and intrusive luxation injuries
- Although it is a chronic and, therefore, very slow process, there is still extensive destruction (resorption) of the cementum and the dentin
- Like inflammatory resorption, replacement resorption is not a self-limiting process
- Requires immediate attention by the practitioner
- Usually a result of severe damage to the periodontium during an avulsion injury
- Bacteria and necrotic pulpal tissue do not seem to play a role in its mechanism of action
- Patients are generally asymptomatic and unaware of the severe destructive nature of this type of resorption

---

* * * * * Clinical Note   * * * * *

This type of resorptive process is generally very slow
and may take months or years to occur.

- Radiographically, replacement resorption is noted for its radio-paque characteristic of bone replacing tooth structure at the same time it is being resorbed by clastic cells
- Can occur along any surface of the root where damage to the periodontium has occurred
- Usually large areas of the tooth are affected and there is no limit to the number of areas or to the size of damage

Idiopathic Root Resorption

- As name implies, a resorptive process without any apparent etiology
- Often seen around the cervical portion of teeth and is some-times referred to as cervical resorption because of its location
- Seen in all tooth groups and in both arches

- In some cases, the affected teeth will have a history of ortho-dontic movement or an internal bleaching procedure months to years prior to the onset of the resorptive process
- Many cases of resorption of this nature are in teeth with seem-ingly vital, normal/healthy, carious-free pulps while others occur in teeth that have been endodontically treated
- Not self-limiting and requires immediate attention

---

* * * * *   Clinical Note   * * * * *

Patient symptoms, when present, are usually periodontal in nature and often related to bleeding of the gingiva or sensitivity of the gingiva during brushing and/or mastication.

II. Management of Root Resorption

A. DIAGNOSIS OF INTERNAL ROOT RESORPTION (Nonperforating)

Clinical Symptoms – Radiographic Findings

- Patients are generally asymptomatic
- The caries and/or restorative history of the involved tooth may be negative, moderate, or quite extensive
- Although there is generally chronic inflammation within the pulp, the tooth usually responds within normal limits to pulp tests

---

* * * * *   Clinical Note   * * * * *

If active resorption is present within the root canal system, then the pulp is necessarily vital. That is, if odontoclasts are resorbing the dentin, vital cells must be present and must have a viable blood supply for nourishment. However, it is also possible for the pulp to become necrotic if the spread of inflam-mation becomes too severe and/or has been long standing, at which time the clastic activity ceases and the defect will get no larger.

- The first evidence of the presence of internal root resorption is usually radiographic

- Often, an incidental diagnosis is made from a complete radiographic series and is then verified with additional periapical and bitewing films (if required)

- The lesion can occur anywhere along the length of the root canal system

- Radiographically, the internal defect has the following characteristics
  - well rounded
  - smooth borders
  - well circumscribed
  - symmetric
  - usually ranges in size from just radiographically perceptible to 2-3 times the size of the root canal
  - the lamina dura and the periodontal ligament space are in tact around the entire root surface

- Regardless of the angle exposed, the radiographic lesion will always remain centered on the root

---

* * * * * Clinical Note * * * * *

The ideal method for verifying a radiographic diagnosis of internal root resorption is accomplished by exposing and comparing two different films of the involved tooth. The first film is taken at a straight-on parallel exposure. The second film should be exposed at a mesial (or distal) angulation (20° to 30° only). If the lesion is truly an internal resorptive defect, the radiolucency of the defect will stay centered on the root in both exposures. If, however, an external resorptive defect or a perforating internal defect is present, the lesion will move off from the center of the tooth in a mesial or distal direction depending upon the angulation exposed and whether the defect is facial or lingual to the canal root system (Buccal Object Rule).

B. DIAGNOSIS OF INTERNAL ROOT RESORPTION (Perforating)

Clinical Symptoms – Radiographic Findings

- Patients are generally asymptomatic; however, they may complain about gingival sensitivity if the perforation has encroached upon the epithelial attachment apparatus

- The restorative history of the tooth is the same as for nonperforating internal resorption

- The tooth usually responds within normal limits to pulp tests, although there is considerably more inflammation because of the perforation

- The radiographic determination for perforating IRR is the same as that for nonperforating IRR

- Radiographically, the perforating IRR has the same radiographic characteristics as nonperforating IRR (see above) with the following exceptions:

  - the lamina dura may be missing and/or the periodontal ligament space may be abnormally widened because of the granulation tissue and inflammation from the perforation site

  - the radiographic lesion may shift off of the center of the root since the perforation may be on the lingual or on the buccal surface of the tooth

---

* * * * *   Clinical Note   * * * * *

In some cases, diagnosis of a perforation can only be verified after the initiation of root canal therapy. Use a calcium hydroxide and barium sulfate mix 1) as a hemostatic agent, 2) as an aid in determining whether the canal is perforated, 3) to determine approximately how large the perforation is, and 4) where on the root surface the perforation occurred. This information is particularly necessary if a surgical approach is anticipated to resolve the defect.

C. Treatment of Internal Root Resorption (Perforating and Nonperforating)

- Once a diagnosis has been made, expedient treatment of internal root resorption is mandatory to prevent the clastic cells from causing additional damage to the radicular structure

- Root canal therapy is required in all cases of internal root resorption in order to prevent additional resorption and to remove inflamed and/or necrotic tissue from within the canal system

- Clean and shape the root canal system thoroughly to prevent necrotic breakdown products from causing future endodontic problems

- The treatment for perforating IRR is slightly different than for teeth without resorptive defects and will be addressed at the end of this section
- Cleaning and shaping with hand or rotary instruments of the root canal should be completed

---

***** **Clinical Note** *****

If the defect is in the coronal 1/3 of the canal, consider opening the orifice of the canal system to a larger than normal size in order to augment the ability to clean the defect both mechanically and with irrigant.

- Copious amounts of 5.25% sodium hypochlorite should be used in order to assist in cleansing the defect where instruments may not be able to penetrate
- Obturation of the root canal should occur once the canal has been completely cleaned and shaped
- In the case of perforating IRR, the defect may cause uncontrollable hemorrhage into the canal system during instrumentation. In this case the following methods may be used to aid in cleaning and shaping
  - Leave sodium hypochlorite in the canal system for several minutes before instrumentation
  - If hemorrhage continues to be a problem, pack calcium hydroxide into the canal system for 7-14 days to obtain hemostasis at the next visit
  - In some cases, surgery is necessary to remove the external granulation tissue before obturation of the canal can commence

Obturation of Nonperforating IRR

- The canal is obturated completely with gutta-percha
- If a warm gutta-percha technique is used, the entire canal system including the defect can be obturated with this method
- If lateral condensation is used, a warm gutta-percha technique will provide a better result for obturating the entire defect

---

***** **Clinical Note** *****

Any acceptable method for obturating the defect with gutta-percha can be used since, once the canal system is obturated, the internal resorptive defect will pose no threat to a successful result.

Obturation of Perforating IRR

- The perforation site will pose potential problems for hemorrhage control and control of the obturating material

THREE APPROACHES FOR TREATMENT OF PERFORATING IRR

1. In some cases the canal and defect can be obturated with an accepted material and method without the need for additional therapy (see obturation of nonperforating IRR)

2. In cases where hemorrhage control is a problem or a nonsurgical approach is desired, the placement of calcium hydroxide for several weeks to several months can be used. This method attempts to heal the defect with a calcific barrier so that surgery is not required. Once the defect has calcified, any obturation method will suffice.

3. In those cases where the canal cannot be obturated and calcium hydroxide therapy was unsuccessful, surgery may have to be performed. This approach is required in order to seal the defect on the outer surface of the root before obturating the canal system.

D. DIAGNOSIS OF EXTERNAL ROOT RESORPTION

- Most external resorption defects are diagnosed based solely on their radiographic appearance

Diagnosis of Inflammatory Root Resorption

- Typically seen as a sequelae to avulsion injures
- Large scooped out (resorbed) areas of tooth structure are replaced by radiolucent granulation/inflammatory tissues
- Tooth usually has multiple areas of defects
- Patients are asymptomatic and unaware of the serious nature of this type of resorptive process
- Inflammatory root resorption is extremely rapid and is able to destroy radicular tooth structure in several weeks
- Pulp is necrotic and does not respond to testing

Treatment of Inflammatory Root Resorption

- Root canal therapy must be initiated as soon as possible after a diagnosis is made

***** **Clinical Note** *****

Remove the necrotic tissue completely from within the root canal system as soon as diagnosis is made to minimize the amount of damage this type of pathosis causes. Copious amounts of 5.25% sodium hypochlorite are mandatory in order to maximize removal of the soft tissue present in the canal system during cleaning and shaping.

- Some clinicians suggest the use of calcium hydroxide as an interappointment medicament to aid in the removal of necrotic tissue and as a bacteriocidal agent within the root canal system

- When calcium hydroxide is used as an interappointment medicament, it should remain in the canal system for several weeks before permanent obturation with gutta-percha and sealer

***** **Clinical Note** *****

There is controversy regarding the use of calcium hydroxide as an interappointment medicament with regard to its efficacy. Proper cleaning of the root canal system with 5.25% sodium hypochlorite will usually prevent any additional resorption from occurring. However, in the absence of proper cleaning and shaping techniques or, in those cases where the clinician may not be able to gain access to the entire canal system (fins and other aberrations within the canal system), calcium hydroxide may be used without negative sequelae.

Diagnosis of Replacement Resorption

- Patients are generally asymptomatic

- Patients typically have a history of an avulsion injury or intrusive luxation injury

- Pathognomonic for replacement resorption is a "wooden-like" sound when a tooth is percussed or a "hollow" type of percussion sound

- There is no mobility in the tooth or extremely little compared to a contralateral tooth

- Pulp is generally nonvital if the etiology is trauma and will not respond to testing

Treatment of Replacement Resorption

- Endodontic therapy is performed if the pulp has been diagnosed as necrotic — this is highly likely after an avulsion or intrusive luxation injury

- Unlike inflammatory resorption, endodontic therapy is not a treatment for replacement resorption

---

* * * * * Clinical Note * * * * *

As of the writing of this Handbook, replacement resorption is an untreatable process. Therefore, warn the patient that in all likelihood, a tooth diagnosed with replacement resorption will be lost eventually.

- Replacement resorption in a young patient with a developing mandible/maxilla will likely cause tooth submergence which may lead to an aesthetic problem with time

- The young patient diagnosed with replacement resorption should be informed of the likelihood of tooth submergence and potential restorative procedures to eliminate

- Because replacement resorption is chronic, although the tooth will likely be lost, the patient will in all probability maintain the tooth for many months to several years

- Older patients generally have a better prognosis with replacement resorption than younger patients

Diagnosis of Idiopathic Resorption

- Tooth has no history of trauma or other etiology for the resorptive process to take place

- Pulp is usually vital and responds normally to testing

- Radiographic evidence of resorbing coronal tooth structure (cervical area) or section of root

  - Depending upon where the resorption is occurring, a radiolucent type of resorptive process similar to the appearance of inflammatory resorption (typical in the cervical portion of the tooth)

  - May get replacement of the tooth structure with bone, similar to replacement resorption (usually highly associated with apical and middle thirds of roots)

Treatment of Idiopathic Resorption

- Because the dental pulp has nothing to do with the resorptive process, root canal therapy is not indicated

- In cases where a surgical approach is possible, the removal of the granulation tissue within the defect has been demonstrated to inhibit the resorptive process

---

***** **Clinical Note** *****

The clinician and patient must be aware that there is a high probability that the resorptive process will return, even though the tissue was removed. It is extremely difficult to remove every bit of granulation tissue in these types of defects. Many resorptive defects wrap around the proximal surfaces of the tooth making access to this tissue almost impossible, thereby, making the return of the resorptive process highly likely.

E. CALCIUM HYDROXIDE

- When mixed for use in resorption cases, can be combined with barium sulfate in a ratio of 6-8:1 (calcium hydroxide:barium sulfate)
- Mixed with barium sulfate and saline, anesthetic, or sterile water
- When used alone or mixed with barium sulfate, should have the consistency of a "clay" mixture of IRM
- Can be introduced into the canal with an amalgam carrier
    - Once in the access opening, a plugger, large gutta-percha cone, or paper point can be used to position material to the desired location
- Proprietary brands can be placed into canal with lentulo spirals
- Should remain in the canal for a minimum of 2-3 months
- Can be used as a diagnostic tool to determine where perforation site is on root surface

FREQUENTLY ASKED QUESTIONS (FAQs)

1. *Is it necessary to use calcium hydroxide in cases of nonperforating internal resorption?*

    Some practitioners like to use it because of its high pH and bacteriocidal effects. However, there is not indication in cases of nonperforating internal resorption to use the medicament since proper cleaning and shaping of canal system with proper obturation will provide a high success rate.

2. *In cases of inflammatory root resorption, how long should calcium hydroxide be left in the canal?*

> A minimum of 2-3 months. After that period of time, it is unlikely that the medicament will be of any additional value. However, if the resorptive process is continuing, then the medicament should be left in the canal until no further evidence of resorption exists.

3. *How often should I change the calcium hydroxide?*

> That depends on how quickly it "washes" out of the canal system. In many cases, especially when barium sulfate and calcium hydroxide are mixed together, it will last up to 6-8 months without having to be changed. The commercial types of calcium hydroxide tend to "wash" out more quickly because they tend to be less viscous.

4. *What's the best type of calcium hydroxide to use?*

> No data supports one brand over another. It's really a function of whether one wants to mix their own or use a proprietary mixture.

Chapter XIV

Apexogenesis and Apexification

APEXOGENESIS & APEXIFICATION

- Apexogenesis and apexification are biologic processes that occur in teeth with incomplete apical formation

- Apexogenesis relates to teeth with retained viable pulp tissue in which this pulp tissue is protected, treated, or encouraged to permit the process of normal root lengthening, root wall thickening, and apical closure

- Apexification relates to teeth with necrotic pulps following carious invasion or trauma

    - Root canal is cleaned and a filling material is placed that will permit a hard tissue barrier to form at the root apex or actually stimulate this formation

A. APEXOGENESIS

- Biologic process of normal root-end formation

- Treatment modality when the pulp has become compromised but retains its viability

- Performed on all permanent teeth

- Treatment of choice, as opposed to root canal treatment, in the immature tooth

- When observing for apical closure radiographically, the mesial and distal root walls will close prior to the buccal and lingual root walls

- Following a successful apexogenesis, root canal treatment may only be required if the pulp exhibits signs or symptoms of inflammation or degeneration, or if the root canal space is required to rebuild the tooth

- With the advent of acid-etching and dentin bonding, the coronal seal of teeth undergoing apexogenesis has been improved, thereby enhancing the quality of the ultimate root formation and a reduced need for further root canal treatment

- If root canal treatment required – usually performed without complications

- See patient for re-examination every 3 months for approximately one year

Clinical Treatment Considerations

- **Trauma and Exposure of Dentinal Tubules**
    - Protect tubules with cavity liner or calcium hydroxide
    - Restore with acid-etched, bonded composite to ensure the coronal seal
    - Pulp should exhibit no symptoms or signs of demise

- **Traumatic, Restorative, or Small Carious Exposure of the Dental Pulp**
    - Pulp capping with calcium hydroxide or MTA (mineral trioxide aggregate)
    - Restore with an acid-etched composite
    - Pulp should exhibit no symptoms or signs of demise

- **Traumatic or Carious Exposure of a Larger Portion of the Coronal Pulp**
    - Pulp may exhibit no signs of inflammation or may have reversible pulpitis
    - Contaminated tissue removed via either a partial pulpotomy or pulpotomy
    - Coronal radicular pulp stump covered with calcium hydroxide or MTA (mineral trioxide aggregate)
    - Bridging of the pulp with dentin desirable to permit the remaining radicular pulp to continue with normal root formation
    - Restore appropriately to ensure a coronal seal

B. APEXIFICATION

- Removal of the necrotic or irreversibly inflamed pulp essential
- Removal occurs to within 1 mm of the incomplete root apex formation
    - Seen radiographically as having either divergent or parallel root walls in the apical third of the developing root
    - Often the root may only be half formed when compared to the adjacent teeth
- Large radiolucency will usually be present when the pulp is necrotic
- Apical extent of the root walls demonstrate a thin, narrow appearance

Clinical Treatment Considerations

- Clean root canal thoroughly
  - Use 2.6% to 5.25% sodium hypochlorite
  - Canal should be free of debris, blood, or pus
- Place either calcium hydroxide or MTA
  (mineral trioxide aggregate)
- Material carried to the apical portion of the root with files or pluggers
- Some forms of calcium hydroxide are injectable
- Calcium hydroxide can be mixed using 6-8 parts of powder with 1 part of barium sulfate powder – liquid is sterile water, saline, or anesthetic solution

---

***** Clinical Note *****

Do not mix with phenolic compounds, such as formocreosol, camphorated paramonochlorophenol, cresatin, or eugenol with calcium hydroxide.

- Can fill canal entirely with calcium hydroxide
  - Canal must be sealed coronally to prevent leakage

***** Clinical Note *****

One of the greatest etiologies for failure of apexification is an inappropriate restoration. Because the patient will likely have the intracanal medicament in place for a minimum of 3 months, a dentin bonding agent and composite (anterior teeth) or amalgam (posterior teeth) restoration is indicated.

- Review case radiographically and clinically every 3 months for 6-24 months
- The calcification that is formed at the apex is porous
  - When determining if an apical barrier has formed, use a size #25 file and probe gently against the barrier
- If no evidence that an apical hard tissue barrier is formed, or if there are patient signs or symptoms, replace calcium hydroxide
- Once a barrier is observed and the patient is asymptomatic, fill root canal with a softened gutta-percha and sealer

- If MTA is placed apically – this is a permanent restoration and should not need future replacement (as recommended by the manufacturer)
  - Long-term clinical and research data is unavailable on these outcomes
- Place permanent restoration following use of MTA

FREQUENTLY ASKED QUESTIONS (FAQs)

1. *What is the anticipated time for apexogenesis to occur?*

   This depends on the degree of root development prior to the challenge to the dental pulp. Follow-up evaluation is necessary every 3 months to ensure normal root development is occurring.

2. *Can an exposed pulp on a tooth with immature apical development receive a direct acid-etched, dentin-bonded restoration without the placement of a pulp-capping material?*

   There are no data to support the placement of an acid-etched, dentin-bonded restoration on a compromised pulp. Available data are scanty and deal primarily with previously unchallenged dental pulp.

3. *Does the calcium hydroxide that is used in the apexification technique need to be replaced on a regular basis?*

   No – replacement is only recommended if there are signs or symptoms of treatment failure, if coronal leakage is detected, or if there is evidence that the calcium hydroxide has "washed out."

4. *What is the best way to obturate the root canal after a successful apexification procedure?*

   A softened gutta-percha technique, such as an injectable technique, can be used. Other techniques include the creation of a custom-fit master gutta-percha cone followed by cold lateral compaction or warm vertical compaction.

5. *Why can't camphorated paramonochlorophenol be mixed with the calcium hydroxide as indicated in the original "Frank Technique" for apexification?*

> The use of phenolic-type liquids promotes severe, long-term tissue damage and chronic inflammation. Tissue regeneration cannot occur in the presence of these types of substances.

6. *Is it necessary to use a different intracanal irrigant in a tooth with immature root development and a necrotic pulp because of potential contact with the periradicular tissues?*

> No — a 2.6% to 5.25% solution of sodium hypochlorite is indicated. This range and type of solution is standard for all root canal treatment.

Chapter XV

Pulpal - Periodontal Interactions

PULPAL – PERIODONTAL INTERACTIONS

- Dental pulp intimately associated with the supporting periodontium

- Unique interchange of inflammatory processes with variable responses on the part of both tissues

- Interchange occurs via multiple anatomical pathways or following therapeutic procedures

- Controversy exists in the dental literature as to mutual interchange of diseases

A. PATHWAYS OF INFLAMMATORY INTERCHANGE

- Apical foramen of the main canal

- Accessory or lateral canals

- Dentinal tubules

- Areas of cemental agenesis

- Resorptive defects

- Tooth cracks or fractures

- Following scaling and/root planing procedures

- Following periodontal/osseous surgical procedures

- Possible bacterial toxin penetration through the cementum in the presence of long-term periodontal disease

- Possible impact of endodontic procedures or endodontic materials

B. IMPACT OF PULPAL INFLAMMATION ON THE PERIODONTIUM

- Process rapid and acute as it extends to the periodontium

- Crestal extension of the disease process in the periodontium occurs, mimicking periodontal disease

- Extension occurs through accessory or lateral canals into the tooth furcation

- Buccal swelling may occur that mimics a periodontal abscess

- Radiographic appearance of the extension into the periodontium (bone loss) usually isolated finding that is not present on other teeth
- Inflammatory movement from the pulp to the periodontium and sequelae documented in dental literature

C. IMPACT OF PERIODONTAL DISEASE ON THE DENTAL PULP

- Process chronic in nature
- Impact enhanced in conjunction with extensive restorative procedures
- Pulp undergoes slow degeneration
- Acceptable or delayed responses to pulp tests
- Radiographic changes in the pulp chamber and canal space often evident
- Degenerative changes evident
  - Include calcification, irregular dentin formation, internal resorption, and small areas of tissue infarction
- Generalized periodontal disease usually present
- Symptoms of pulpal disease absent unless an acute state of inflammation present
- Inflammatory impact of periodontal disease and sequelae controversial when the dental literature reviewed

D. REASONS FOR CONTROVERSIES IN THE PULPAL – PERIODONTAL INTERCHANGE

- Most studies are observational only
- Extent of pulpal degeneration prior to the periodontal disease state not determined
- Little mention of previous periodontal treatment when trying to establish a relationship for the impact of periodontal disease on the pulp
- Periodontally normal teeth not included in the study
- Minimal to no inclusion of age-matched teeth for comparison
- Minimal correlation of bacterial species and their toxins from one tissue to the other
- Variations in anatomical pathways of communication exist

- Animal species that serve as the basis for the investigations vary
- Validity of data extrapolation among species questionable

E. CLASSIFICATION

- Clinical purposes of diagnosis and case management – 6 categories
    - Primary pulpal disease
    - Primary pulpal disease with secondary periodontal disease
    - Primary periodontal disease
    - Primary periodontal disease with secondary pulpal disease
    - Combined pulpal – periodontal disease states
    - Concomitant pulpal – periodontal disease states

PRIMARY PULPAL DISEASE

- Clinical diagnosis indicates an irreversible pulpitis or a necrotic pulp
- Often a rapid onset
- In molar teeth, the furcation area may appear radiographically to have significant bone loss
- Minimal to no calculus present and no evidence of generalized or advance periodontitis
- Tooth mobile or exhibit a narrow channel sinus tract
- Swelling present in the attached gingiva and the tooth sore to biting or chewing

---

***** **Clinical Note** *****

When this diagnosis is determined, root canal treatment only is indicated. Do not curette furcation region or use caustic, inflammatory medicaments in the pulp chamber.

PRIMARY PULPAL DISEASE WITH SECONDARY PERIODONTAL DISEASE

- Clinical diagnosis indicates an irreversible pulpitis or a necrotic pulp
- Evidence for the presence of periodontal disease, with vertical bone loss, inflamed soft tissues, and calculus
- Radiographic changes in the pulpal space visible with linear or isolated calcific changes

***** **Clinical Note** *****

When this diagnosis is determined, root canal treatment and periodontal treatment are indicated. Simultaneous management is preferable. Prognosis for resolution is dependent on the ability to treat both disease entities successfully.

PRIMARY PERIODONTAL DISEASE

– Clinical and radiographic assessments indicate generalized, moderate to deep bony pockets

– Diffuse gingival inflammation

– Asymptomatic patient and pulp responds to testing within normal limits

***** **Clinical Note** *****

Treatment is limited to periodontal therapy only with the prognosis dependent on the ability to remove the causative factors and the patient's ability to achieve meticulous self-care practices.

PRIMARY PERIODONTAL DISEASE WITH SECONDARY PULPAL DISEASE

– Clinical and radiographic assessments indicate broad-based probings, vertical, and possible apical or lateral bone loss

– Symptomatic pulpitis or necrotic pulp

– Symptoms acute and history of previous, extensive periodontal treatment

– Tooth often has or needs extensive restoration

***** **Clinical Note** *****

Successful treatment is dependent on the removal of the causative factors for periodontal disease and the patient's ability to achieve meticulous self-care practices once the root canal treatment has been performed.

COMBINED PULPAL AND PERIODONTAL DISEASE

- Clinical and radiographic assessments indicate infrabony periodontal pocket

- Communication with an isolated periradicular lesion of pulpal origin

- Pulp testing indicates a necrotic pulp

- Probing may reveal vertical fracture

- Symptoms may be acute or chronic

***** Clinical Note *****

Perform root canal treatment first to manage acute symptoms, if any. Treat periodontally concomitantly. Prognosis is better if the extension of the pulpal disease impacts on existing periodontal disease and if the combined process has been short-term.

CONCOMITANT PULPAL AND PERIODONTAL DISEASE

- Clinical and radiographic assessments indicate disease processes exist independent of each other

- Broad-based probings present

- Presence of a necrotic pulp (due to caries, extensive restorations, or trauma)

- If symptoms present, usually due to pulpal inflammation

***** Clinical Note *****

If symptoms are present, treat cause first. If not, both root canal treatment and periodontal treatment must be performed concomitantly. The prognosis is dependent on the removal of all causative factors.

F. SURGICAL ROOT OR TOOTH RESECTIONS

(See Chapter XXI for details on these procedures)

***** **Clinical Note** *****

The classifications discussed above refer only to the interchange of disease processes in the presence of an inflamed
dental pulp, a necrotic dental pulp, and the multiple stages
of periodontal disease. These are pulpal-periodontal interactions or relationships and must be understood for a
proper differential diagnosis and treatment planning.
Other interactions occur that are more accurately
referred to as endodontic-periodontic problems.
These usually occur after root canal treatment
has been performed, such as vertical fractures,
evidence of a root perforation, coronal
leakage, and its impact on the periodontium in what appears to be
quality root canal treatment.

FREQUENTLY ASKED QUESTIONS (FAQs)

1. *Should teeth be pulp tested prior to periodontal treatment?*

    Yes, prior to treatment and periodically after periodontal
    treatment, especially if restorative procedures are planned.

2. *Will all teeth that have extensive periodontal disease or
   periodontal treatment require root canal treatment?*

    No — treatment will be required only if significant changes
    occur in the health of the dental pulp. Evidence for these
    changes may take months to years – or may not occur at all.

3. *If a periodontally involved tooth needs a hemisection or
   root resection (amputation), is root canal treatment necessary?*

    The dental literature provides a number of case reports that
    cite evidence for short-term success with "vital resections."
    Long-term success is poor and valid prognostic data are
    unavailable. Root canal treatment is recommended in all
    cases – and when possible, prior to the resective procedure.

4. **Does an acute periradicular lesion with soft tissue swelling require periodontal treatment?**

No — the cause of the problem is entirely from the dental pulp, only endodontic treatment is necessary.

5. **Does rapid furcation bone loss secondary to an acute periradicular lesion require periodontal curettage?**

No — the rapid breakdown of the bone in the furcation is due primarily to the coronal extension of the periradicular lesion, or the movement of toxins from the acute inflammatory process in the dental pulp chamber into the furcation region. Root canal treatment only is indicated.

6. **Does a chronic draining sinus tract through the gingival sulcus require periodontal treatment?**

A draining sinus tract indicates that the pulp is likely necrotic. There, root canal treatment is indicated. Periodontal treatment may be indicated after the root canal treatment if the sinus tract fails to heal, indicating a secondary periodontal problem. This can often be identified if there is calculus present in the defect created by the sinus tract.

7. **Can pulp tests help to establish the status of the supporting periodontium?**

Pulp tests can only establish the responsiveness of the dental pulp.

8. **On a tooth with periodontal disease and a symptomatic pulp, does it make any difference if the two processes are related?**

No — both root canal treatment and periodontal therapy are necessary for an optimal prognosis.

9. **How can probings be used to indicate whether pulpal or periodontal disease exists?**

Narrow channel probings usually indicate 1) the presence of a draining sinus tract of pulpal origin that has penetrated into the gingival sulcus; or, 2) the possible presence of a vertical fracture. Note the vertical fracture does not provide a pulpal diagnosis; it only indicates the presence of a tooth – bone – soft tissue defect. The signs, symptoms, and evaluative testing of the dental pulp will still dictate the pulpal diagnosis.

Chapter XVI

Cracked & Fractured Teeth

CRACKED & FRACTURED TEETH

- Factors that predispose to cracks and fractures are often not controllable
- Clinical detection of fractures can be difficult
- Patient symptoms are often bizarre and difficult to reproduce
- Patient symptoms can mimic other diagnoses
- Management is dependent on a unique set of treatment variables

A. CLASSIFICATION

- Craze lines
- Fractured cusps
- Cracked teeth
- Fractured teeth
- Vertical root fractures

B. RESTORATIVE FACTORS THAT CONTRIBUTE TO CRACKED OR FRACTURED TEETH

- Soft gold inlay
- Large undermining amalgams
- Excessive removal of tooth structure
- Reinforcing pins
- Intraradicular posts/dowels
- Insertion pressures with post cementation
- Failure to restore properly endodontically-treated teeth (see Chapter XVII)
- Improper occlusal adjustments

C. ENDODONTIC FACTORS THAT CONTRIBUTE TO CRACKED OR FRACTURED TEETH

- Excessive canal shaping and removal of sound dentin

- Excessive compaction forces during obturation
- Wedging of filling materials and instruments
- Excessive use of straight rotary instruments (eg, Peeso reamers/Gates Glidden burs)

D. MISCELLANEOUS FACTORS THAT CONTRIBUTE TO CRACKED OR FRACTURED TEETH

- Periodontal disease with significant bone loss
- Pathologic entities
- Traumatic occlusion – bruxism
- Anterior open bites – posterior cross bites
- Anatomical tooth form
- Tooth abrasion or erosion

E. SUBJECTIVE FINDINGS WITH CRACKED OR FRACTURED TEETH

- Often, there is sustained pain during biting
- Pain only upon release of biting is also found

---

* * * * *   **Clinical Note**   * * * * *

Pathognomonic for "cracked tooth syndrome" is pain/sensitivity upon release of mastication forces. Many endodontic diagnoses have mastication sensitivity upon closure, but cracked tooth syndrome is specific with sensitivity upon release (opening) of pressure on an object.

- Occasional, momentary, sharp pain during mastication
- Sensitivity to thermal changes may be evident
- Persistent dull pain after eating in the later stages

```
*****    Clinical Note    *****
```

Not all cracked teeth require root canal therapy. Often a large restoration that protects the fractured tooth segment is appropriate. In some cases, removal of the fractured segment is required. However, if the fracture extends along the long axis of the tooth toward the pulp, either "chasing" the fracture until it is removed, or cuspal coverage (onlay or crown) is indicated.

F. OBJECTIVE FINDINGS WITH CRACKED OR FRACTURED TEETH

- Pain to selective percussion on specific tooth margins or cusps

- Generalized discomfort to percussion

- Presence of crazes, cracks or fracture lines on the facial or lingual surfaces or marginal ridges

- Significant gaps between old restorations and tooth structure

- Cracked restorations

- Narrow channel sinus tracts along the periodontium

- Radiographic evidence of thickened PDL space

- Diffuse longitudinal radiolucencies

- Radiolucent fracture line with or without segment separation

- Radiopaque lines visible in the treated root canal

- Teeth commonly fractured include mandibular molars and maxillary premolars

G. TREATMENT MAY BE REQUIRED TO MAKE A DIAGNOSIS

- Angled radiographs

- Biting or percussion testing

- Removal of restorations, including crowns and bridges

- Staining of the tooth structure with methylene blue

- Fiber optic disclosure of fracture lines

- Laser pointer light

- Surgical exposure to identify root fractures

H. TREATMENT OPTIONS

- **CRAZE LINES**
  - No treatment necessary
  - Note presence and location of lines
  - Advise patient

- **FRACTURED CUSPS**
  - Patient usually has symptoms
  - Symptoms rarely indicate an irreversible pulpitis
  - Treat as reversible pulpitis
  - Identify offending cusp; remove and restore
  - If symptoms persist, do root canal treatment

- **CRACKED TEETH**
  - Painful to bite and often cold
  - Segments are not mobile – pulp irreversibly damaged
  - Root canal treatment indicated
  - Full coverage restoration
  - If crack progresses, tooth may be lost

- **FRACTURED TEETH**
  - Usually two distinct, separable segments
  - Pain present on mastication and periodontium is sore
  - Extraction usually indicated
  - Some cases amenable to endodontic, periodontic, ortho-
    dontic, and restorative management if a viable segment of
    the tooth can be maintained

- **VERTICAL ROOT FRACTURES**
  - Fracture begins in the root
  - Often occurs in teeth with previous root canal treatment
  - More common in teeth with posts or very large restorations
  - Symptoms and signs may be minimal
  - Narrow channel sinus tract or probing present
  - Extraction – root resection – tooth resection (see Chapter
    XXI)

FREQUENTLY ASKED QUESTIONS (FAQs)

1. *How can I distinguish a sinus tract of pulpal origin from one that is from a vertical fracture and a periodontal pocket?*

   Periodontal pockets are broad-based and the probe can move laterally when at its depth in the sulcus. Patient symptoms will also tend to indicate whether the pulp is affected. Sinus tracts that trace up the sulcus can occur, but are rare. Patients will also exhibit pain to selective percussion and biting with vertical fractures. Ultimate determination can be done, if necessary, with a surgical entry.

2. *When is a cracked tooth doomed to extraction?*

   When the periodontium has been challenged by the extent of the crack. For example, if the crack line in a mandibular molar runs down both marginal ridges and across the floor of the chamber, extraction is indicated. If limited to the ridges, it is possible to do root canal treatment and bond the coronal portion of the tooth – with a guarded prognosis.

Restoration of the Endodontically-Treated Tooth

RESTORATION OF THE ENDODONTICALLY-TREATED TOOTH

- Controversial because of the lack of scientific support for the various treatment procedures recommended

- Significant increase in the supporting scientific data in past 20 years

- New paradigm has emerged in the view of the restorative needs of an endodontically-treated tooth

A. PHYSICAL, ARCHITECTURAL, BIOCHEMICAL, & BIOCHEMICAL CHANGES IN TOOTH STRUCTURE FOLLOWING ROOT CANAL TREATMENT

- Important considerations in tooth structure

  - Modulus of elasticity

  - Compressive and tensile strength

  - Ductility, hardness, and toughness

  - Moisture loss and brittleness

  - Architectural changes

  - Changes in collagen structure

- Endodontically-treated teeth do not experience a significant loss of moisture following root treatment

- Loss of significant portions of the tooth structure, such as marginal ridges and cuspal architecture, play a significant role in the weakening of the root-filled tooth

- 30% of the ultimate tensile strength of the dentin provided by collagen

  - Collagen undergoes significant changes in strength after root canal treatment

- Evaluation of the biomechanical properties of endodontically-treated teeth indicate that they do not become brittle

---

***** **Clinical Note** *****

Teeth do not fracture because they become "brittle." This term
is actually a misnomer. The moisture content that is lost in
a tooth after root canal therapy is minimal and does
not contribute significantly to fracture.

- Retention of sound dentin, a major factor in the retained
  strength of the endodontically-treated tooth

- All endodontically-treated teeth do not need a post, core and
  crown – but should be evaluated as to the factors below

***** **Clinical Note** *****

Too often, posts are placed routinely in endodontically-treated
teeth with the intent of "strengthening the tooth." Posts
will act only as a device to hold the restorative core
in place and will not add appreciably any
strength to the tooth.

B. ANATOMICAL VARIATIONS IN TOOTH STRUCTURE OF IMPORTANCE

- Internal and external root anatomy
- Cross section of root walls
- Root wall thickness
- Curvatures and tapers
- Proximal invaginations

C. CLINICAL FACTORS THAT AFFECT THE RESTORATION OF ENDODONTICALLY-TREATED TEETH

- Occlusion and function
- Tooth position in the arch
- Periodontal status
- Prosthetic needs
- Remaining tooth structure
- Root morphology and integrity
- Economics

D. POST TYPES

- **CUSTOM CAST POSTS**
  - Difficult to make
  - Laboratory shortcomings
  - Cost
  - Interim restoration may be demanding
  - When used properly, prefabricated posts acceptable

- **PREFABRICATED POSTS**
  - Passive retention – depend on proximity to the walls and the adherence of the cement
  - Active retention – depend on the dentin engagement and the cement as a secondary issue

- **TYPES OF PREFABRICATED POSTS**
  - Tapered, smooth – have low retention; little or no installation stresses; wedging effect during function
  - Parallel, serrated – have higher retention; little or no installation stresses; functional stress uniformly distributed via the cement layer
  - Tapered, self-threading screw type – intermediate retention; high-wedging stresses during installation; potential high stresses during function
  - Parallel, threaded – high retention; low installation stresses after counter rotation; low functional stresses
  - Parallel, serrated, tapered end – have higher retention; little or no installation stresses; wedging effect at apex during function

E. CONSIDERATIONS IN THE CEMENTATION OF POSTS IN TEETH

- Zinc phosphate acceptable when mixed properly
- Smear layer should be removed
- Use unfilled resins
- Use newer post-cementing media designed with enhanced compressive and tensile strengths
- Use bonding agents/systems

F. COMPELLING REASONS FOR NOT PLACING A POST IN ENDODONTICALLY-TREATED TEETH

- Need to remove additional sound tooth structure
- No effective root strengthening with the post
- Potential for fractures during installation
- Potential for fracture during mastication
- Periodontal bone loss
- Adverse root morphology
- Stress patterns in the root are altered when posts are placed

G. CORE BUILDUPS – MATERIALS

- Bonded amalgams and composites acceptable
- Use specific composites designated as core materials (eg, Ti-Core, Core Paste)
- Do not use glass ionomers as core materials
- Cores must be on sound tooth structure
- At least 1.5-2.0 mm of sound dentin must be available below the core material for the crown margin
- The biologic width must not be violated

H. CLINICAL GUIDELINES FOR RESTORING ENDODONTICALLY-TREATED TEETH

- Cusps of posterior teeth should be covered
- Resist placement of posts in mesial roots of mandibular molars and buccal roots of maxillary molars
- Large round posts should not be placed in the distal roots of mandibular molars or the palatal roots of maxillary molars
- Placement of posts in roots unsupported by bone results in adverse concentration of forces a the end of the post
- Primary role of post is to assist in core retention
- Increases in post size and diameter do not increase retention
- Carbon fiber posts have not had sufficient evaluation to warrant their routine use
- If a post is used it should not be greater that 1/3 of the entire root width in all dimensions

***** **Clinical Note** *****

The restoration of endodontically-treated teeth requires an in-depth assessment of multiple factors before determining the best treatment plan. When finally restored, the tooth must function as a single unit and be subjected to minimal occlusal forces to prevent the dislodgement of the post, core, and crown. Failure generally occurs because of open crown margins, coronal leakage, and dislodgement of the post, core or crown, or tooth/root fracture.

FREQUENTLY ASKED QUESTIONS (FAQs)

1. *Why can't glass ionomers be used for core buildups?*

    Glass ionomers do not have the internal strength necessary to serve as a core. If they are surrounded completely by sound tooth structure, they may be able to suffice in nonload-bearing areas of the mouth.

2. *What can be done to ensure proper crown margins when the decayed margin is deep and the core material is below the gingival tissue?*

    In these circumstances, surgical crown lengthening should be treatment planned at the time of or before the root canal therapy.

3. *What is the best prefabricated post system?*

    The one that provides the best restoration for the tooth in question without compromising tooth structure and function.

4. *Because of their retention, aren't screw posts the best?*

    Screw posts can provide a good restoration provided that 1) they are not tapered and create a wedging effect during placement or function; 2) that the grooves in the root for the threads are created before cementation; 3) they are counter rotated 1/2 to 1/4 turn after placement; and 4) they are used only to assist in core retention.

Chapter XVIII

Nonsurgical Retreatment

NONSURGICAL RETREATMENT

A. TYPICAL REASONS FOR FAILURE OF NONSURGICAL ROOT CANAL TREATMENT

- Main reason for failure is improper cleaning of the root canal system and improper seal

- Coronal leakage

- Broken instruments within canals

***** **Clinical Note** *****

Broken instruments within the canal system do not necessarily cause failure of root canal treatment. It is a function of how much cleaning and shaping was completed before the instrument broke within the canal system. If the canal system has been instrumented at least to a #25 K file, then the likelihood of success is very high. However, if the canal system was not adequately cleaned, and an instrument is now preventing the completion of debridement, then the likelihood of failure is high.

- Paste fills

- Improper obturation of the canal system

- Leakage of saliva from interappointment loss of temporary and failure to reinstrument and reclean the canal system before obturation

- Failure to recognize additional canals within the root canal system

    - Typically mandibular molar distal canals, maxillary MB/MP canals (see Chapter II)

- Lost or leaking permanent restoration

- Inability to negotiate and instrument calcified canals

B. ARMAMENTARIUM AND METHODS SPECIFIC TO THE MATERIAL IN THE ROOT CANAL FOR RETREATMENT

- Numerous devices are available for retreatment of most obturation materials
- Correct armamentarium is a function of the type of obturation material within the canal system

Gutta-Percha Removal

- Easiest and most expedient is with heat

***** **Clinical Note** *****

Once bulk of gutta-percha (usually coronal half of canal) has been removed with a heat instrument, a hedström file (minimum size #25) can be twisted into the remaining gutta-percha and the remaining material is easily removed in one pass.

- Schilder OP instrument
- Pluggers and spreaders are contraindicated because they are not heat tempered and will break after several uses
- Peeso reamers

***** **Clinical Note** *****

Extreme caution should be exercised whenever Peeso reamers are used for removal of canal obturation materials. These devices will easily go off track and begin to remove dentin instead of maintaining themselves within the canal. Perforation can easily occur especially in curved canals.

- Files
- Glick #2 or #1 heat Instrument

Solvents

- Solvents should be placed into pulp chamber and carried into the canal system with files or other instruments
- Solvents should be left within the chamber for several minutes to allow time for softening of the obturation material
- Chloroform

- White Pine Oil
- Eucalyptol
- Rectified Turpentine
- Xylol
- Pine Needle Oil
- Halothane
- Oil of Melaleuca

***** Clinical Note *****

Too much solvent, especially in the apical third of the canal,
will cause dissolution of the gutta-percha. This will
often result in a significant amount of gutta-percha
to be pushed outside the canal system.

- When files or other instruments are used to remove gutta-
  percha, ledging and blockage of the canal can occur with
  improper use

Retrieval of Small Metallic Objects
(Silver Points, Broken Files, Gates Glidden Burs)

- Spoon excavators
  - Can be modified by placing a "V" notch into the spoon so
    that it grips the metallic object more securely
- Explorers
- Gates Glidden Burs are designed to break at the top of the
  shank, if the head of this bur breaks within the canal, it is
  virtually impossible to remove

Silver Point Retrievers

  - Modified hemostats
  - Steiglitz forceps
  - Modified forceps
  - Peet splinter forceps
  - Hartmen mosquito forceps

Masserann Kit

  - Very expensive
  - Very versatile
  - Usually required cutting of some tooth structure

- Kit has tubular trephining burs to cut around metallic object
- Usually not indicated in curved or dilacerated canal systems

Ultrasonic Devices

- Excellent method for removing silver points and posts
- Place ultrasonic tip directly on metallic object and leave in place until object loosens
- Must be careful with these devices when removing silver points, as too high a frequency will cause silver point to break or "dissolve"

---

* * * * *   Clinical Note   * * * * *

If ultrasonic tip cannot be placed directly on object, use an explorer tip or other instrument to contact metallic object and place ultrasonic tip on that instrument to transfer ultrasonic waves.

Twisted Hedström File Technique

- Place three #20-#25 (largest possible) hedström files into the canal system and twist files to wrap around metallic object
- Once files are secure around object, grab files with hemostat and remove slowly
- Often a mirror handle can be placed on tooth to provide leverage and control of hemostat

---

* * * * *   Clinical Note   * * * * *

One of biggest mistakes made during removal of silver points is inadvertent removal of coronal part of silver point within the pulp chamber. This occurs because the silver point is often embedded in the amalgam core or zinc phosphate core within the pulp chamber. During removal of the core material, the silver points are unnoticed and removed with restoration. Once the silver points are noted, then judicious removal of the core material without disturbing the points should be exercised.

Retrieval of Large Metallic Objects (Posts)

- Most posts can be removed easily with ultrasonic devices

- Important to remove all core material, cements, composites, etc, around the post before using ultrasonic

- Core materials have a dampening effect on the ultrasonic instrument and loss of frequency results in longer usage time

  - "Special Bur" (Maillefer) and "Muller Bur" (Hager & Meisinger) are excellent for channeling down along the post

Post Removal Systems

  - Thomas Post Removal System
  - Masserann Kit
  - Brassler Post Remover
  - SS White Post Remover

- Do not attempt to remove post until it demonstrates some mobility within the canal system

- Premature attempts at removing post will often result in fractured tooth structure and split roots

- Virtually every post can be removed with the ultrasonic devices on the market

---

***** **Clinical Note** *****

The key to successful removal of any object within the canal system is patience. With the advent of ultrasonic devices now in the 20-30,000 HZ range, virtually every object can be removed from the canal system. However, both the practitioner and the patient must realize that it often takes 30 minutes to well over an hour of ultrasonic vibrations on a well-seated post before mobility will occur.

C. CLINICAL ASPECTS OF NONSURGICAL RETREATMENT

- Nonsurgical retreatment is often technically more difficult than the original root canal

---

***** **Clinical Note** *****

Multiple errors can occur during retreatment which include perforations while attempting to locate broken instruments and inadvertent loss of critical tooth structure. Ledging during attempts to regain length commonly occurs because of inadequate removal of original obturation material.

- Patients typically have a greater postoperative flare-up rate after retreatment than with conventional first-time treatment

- During most retreatment procedures, material is inadvertently pushed out of the apex (in patent cases) that causes additional postoperative symptoms

- Asymptomatic patients should always be warned that retreatment procedures often cause several days of discomfort and potential swelling and other complications

- Success rates for retreatment are significantly lower than first-time root canal treatment

- If canal blockage is noted or anticipated before retreatment begins, patients should be informed that the prognosis is guarded

- It is imperative to clean and shape the root canal system thoroughly during retreatment procedures

- Sodium hypochlorite (full strength or 50% dilution) should always be used during the cleaning and shaping phase of retreatment

- Antibiotics are not indicated routinely during retreatment procedures

FREQUENTLY ASKED QUESTIONS (FAQs)

1. *Is retreatment or surgery the most predictable procedure?*

   Although surgery would always seem to be the most predictable procedure for the patient, the main reason for failure of surgical endodontics is inadequately cleaned canal systems. Therefore, if possible, retreatment should always be performed before any surgical intervention.

2. *Why are success rates lower for retreatment than for first-time therapy?*

   Although success rates are high for retreatment procedures, they are significantly lower because of the multiple problems that cause the initial failure of the case. If the case has been inadequately cleaned and shaped, and subsequently a file breaks in a canal, then the likelihood of a successful retreatment is very low. If the original canal was blocked during the cleaning and shaping process, the likelihood of getting further into the canal is significantly lowered. However, if during retreatment an additional canal is discovered, then the case will have a high success rate.

3. *Why do patients have a high flare-up rate after retreatment?*

There is a high probability that necrotic debris and obturation material will be pushed through a patent apex during any retreatment procedure. This material will often cause mastication sensitivity, minor swelling, and generalized throbbing pain in the affected area. Most often, nonsteroidal analgesics are sufficient to manage the patient.

Chapter XIX

Bleaching in Endodontics

BLEACHING IN ENDODONTICS

- Bleaching of teeth, vital and nonvital, is primarily indicated for cosmetic purposes

A. TYPES OF STAINING

Intrinsic Staining (Vital Pulps)

- – Usually due to systemic drugs
- – Tetracyclines that alter the color of the dentin
- Due to drug interference with tooth development, such as fluorosis
  - – Affects the quality of the enamel matrix
- Intrinsic staining (nonvital pulps) – due to a myriad of causes
  - – Necrotic pulp
  - – Hemosiderin pigment
  - – Calcific metamorphosis from trauma
  - – Developmental defects
  - – Root canal filling materials and sealer-cements (silver cones, silver-staining sealers)
  - – Pulp tissue remnants
  - – Intracanal medicaments
  - – Intracanal restorations (amalgams)
  - – Corrosion of fillings

Extrinsic Staining (Both Vital and Nonvital Pulp)

- – Poor oral hygiene
- – Coffee and tea
- – Foods
- – Tobacco products

***** **Clinical Note** *****

Identify the cause of the staining before treatment planning its
management. Some stains cannot be modified and others
can only be altered slightly. This determination will
ultimately direct the treatment plan
for the patient.

B. BLEACHING OF VITAL TEETH

- Known as "vital bleaching" – application of an oxidizer to the enamel surface of a tooth with a vital pulp

- Subjected to multiple variables such as location and cause of stain

- If stain in dentin, success limited

- If stain in enamel, greater success anticipated

C. MATERIALS & TECHNIQUES – VITAL TEETH

- For intrinsic stains, in-office requires a 30% hydrogen peroxide application with additional heat provided to the enamel surface

  - Temperatures in the range of 125°F to 142°F

- Isolate teeth from gingival tissues

- Take photographs before starting with subsequent photographs taken to evaluate progress

- Patient application of 10% carbamide peroxide gel in a custom-fitted tray for home use

- Tray with bleaching gel used during the evening hours for 6-8 hours – "nightguard vital bleaching"

- Nightguard bleaching approximately 95% effective when stain not due to tetracycline – can modify some tetracycline staining

- Slight morphological changes in the enamel noted with the vital bleaching gels

- Longevity of success varies

- Side effects include thermal tooth sensitivity and gingival irritation, tooth pain, sore throat, tingling of the tissues, and headaches

- Superficial extrinsic stains more amenable to bleaching – dependent on type and depth of stain

- Bleaching of extrinsic stains may require 18% hydrochloric acid mixed in a pumice paste

- Paste burnished into the enamel surface for 5-10 sections

  - Rinse with water

  - Repeat as necessary

- – Neutralize with a solution of sodium bicarbonate and water
- Alternative – apply the McInnes Technique
    - 30% hydrogen peroxide mixed with 36% hydrochloride acid and a small amount of diethyl ether
    - Applied for 1-2 minutes with cotton applicators
    - Smooth surface with fine-grit disks
    - Repeat several times
- Bleaching of teeth with vital pulps may include root canal treatment followed by bleaching of the now, nonvital tooth from within

---

* * * * *   Clinical Note   * * * * *

Some teeth develop acute irreversible pulpitis following the use of the vital bleaching techniques with carbamide peroxide.

D. MATERIALS & TECHNIQUES – NONVITAL TEETH

- Nonvital bleaching techniques – two categories
    - Thermocatalytic
    - Walking bleach techniques
- Materials
    - Hydrogen peroxide (30%)
    - Sodium perborate
    - Sodium hypochlorite in some cases
- Thermocatalytic
    - Placement of an oxidizing chemical (30% hydrogen peroxide) in the pulp chamber
    - Application of heat, such as heat lamp, heated instrument, or electric heating devices
    - Ultraviolet light application used by some to replace the heat
    - Protect gingival tissues with petroleum jelly
    - Place a rubber dam
    - Access the pulp chamber
    - Cervical area over the root filling sealed with zinc phosphate or zinc oxide-eugenol cement prior to placement of chemicals and heat
    - Place chemical(s) with a cotton pellet

- Apply heat source against or near the pellet, driving the oxygen into the dentin tubules

---

***** **Clinical Note** *****

If the cervical area is not sealed, the bleaching chemical may penetrate patent dentinal tubules in this area and stimulate cervical resorptive response. (See Chapter XIII)

- Walking bleach
  - Rubber dam isolation
  - Remove a thin layer of dentin internally along the facial aspect of the endodontic access cavity
    - Removes some of the stained dentin and creates a fresh smear layer than can be removed prior to bleaching
  - Remove all canal-obturating materials just below the gingival margin
  - Place thin layer of cement (zinc oxide-eugenol or zinc phosphate) over coronal portion of the root filling
  - Etch internal surface lightly to remove the smear layer
  - Place a paste of sodium perborate and hydrogen peroxide in the chamber
  - Seal chamber with a thick mix of zinc oxide-eugenol without intervening cotton pellet
  - See patient within one week
  - Reapply paste if necessary
  - Small amount of color change can be achieved, but is sufficient to satisfy the patient

---

***** **Clinical Note** *****

Failure to place a seal over the root canal filling material has resulted in reports of severe pain during or following the walking bleaching procedure. Oxygen can penetrate along even a good root canal filling into the peri-radicular tissues. Likewise, if the cervical area is not sealed, the bleaching chemical may penetrate patent dentinal tubules in this area and stimulate cervical resorptive response.
(See Chapter XIII)

FREQUENTLY ASKED QUESTIONS (FAQs)

1. *What can I do after nightguard vital bleaching results in a sensitive tooth or teeth?*

   The patient can generally manage tooth sensitivity by brushing with a potassium nitrate-containing toothpaste or by applying fluoride in the same tray that was used for the beaching.

2. *What do I do when the patient has veneers and the dark color of the tooth changes the apparent color of the veneers?*

   A 10% carbamide peroxide gel in a custom fit tray can change the color of the underlying tooth structure.

3. *If the tooth staining that is present has not been removed successfully by vital bleaching techniques, should devitalization of the pulp followed by nonvital bleaching be the treatment of choice?*

   Preferably, a dental pulp that has exhibited no adverse symptoms or signs of degeneration should not be devitalized, although the patient can be given the option of this procedure, veneers, or full porcelain crowns.

Chapter XX

Nonsurgical Endodontic Treatment for Pediatric Patients

NONSURGICAL ENDODONTIC TREATMENT FOR PEDIATRIC PATIENTS

A. MORPHOLOGY OF PRIMARY TEETH

- Pulp chamber is higher occlusally than in permanent teeth

- Shape of pulp chamber is similar to permanent teeth except that it is generally larger in all dimensions

- Soft tissue of pulp is similar to permanent teeth

- Pulp horns are generally higher in primary teeth and, therefore, more subject to insult

- Enamel and dentin is generally thinner in primary teeth

- Root anatomy in primary teeth is significantly different than in permanent teeth

- Presence of multiple lateral and accessory canals in primary teeth

B. PULPAL PATHOSIS AND VITAL PULP MANAGEMENT

Pulpal Diagnosis

- Diagnosis is difficult in primary teeth because of unreliability of some diagnostic tests

- Must rely primarily on radiographs, patient symptoms, and clinical tests

- Diagnosis based on patient symptoms is similar as in permanent teeth

    - History of spontaneous pain-irreversible pulpitis or necrotic pulp

    - Percussion sensitivity-irreversible pulpitis or necrotic pulp

    - Mastication pain-reversible, irreversible, or necrotic pulp

    - Palpation sensitivity-irreversible or necrotic pulp

    - Sensitivity to cold air, sweets, or liquids-reversible or irreversible pulp

- – Generally agreed that electric pulp tests and thermal tests are unreliable in primary teeth
- Radiographic evidence of pulpal pathosis
  - – Radiolucent area on coronal tooth structure
  - – Evidence of internal resorptive areas in pulp chamber or in root canal system
  - – Periradicular changes in surrounding bone like widening of PDL, loss of lamina dura, or radiolucent area(s) present
  - – Furcation areas often demonstrate first evidence of pathosis in primary teeth
  - – Evidence of external root resorption
- Reversible, irreversible, and necrotic pulps in primary teeth can be treated usually with some form of endodontic therapy

Direct Pulp-Capping Therapy

- Defined as a treatment of exposed pulpal tissue due to caries, iatrogenic reasons, or trauma with a material or medicament in order to maintain pulpal vitality
- Purpose of Direct Pulp Cap
  - – Preserve vitality of the pulp
  - – Remove infected and affected dentin
  - – Maintain space for permanent tooth eruption
  - – Maintain support and function of primary tooth
- Critical to prevent salivary contaminants from entering exposure site (use of rubber dam essential)
- Relatively high degree of success with technique
- Contraindicated when signs (clinical or radiographic) and/or symptoms indicate irreversible pulpitis is present
  - – Radiographic evidence of periradicular pathosis
  - – Spontaneous pain from tooth
  - – Sinus tract present/soft tissue swelling
  - – Percussion sensitivity
  - – Absence of frank hemorrhage from exposure site
  - – Severe and/or lingering pain from thermal tests
  - – Inability to control hemorrhage from exposure site
- Controversial procedure among some clinicians as to its clinical value in lieu of other types of procedures available

PULP-CAPPING MATERIALS

- Calcium hydroxide (most popular)
  - Commercial brands and mixed powder are equal in efficacy
  - Calcium ion from medicament does not contribute to bridging of dentin
- Zinc oxide
- Amalgam
- Tricalcium phosphate
- Isobutyl cyanoacrylate
- Collagen
- 4-META
- Antibiotics
- Corticosteroids
- Astringents
- Formocresol

DIRECT PULP-CAPPING TECHNIQUE

- Isolation with rubber dam
- Carious dentin is removed completely
- Exposure is rinsed gently with saline or sterile solution (anesthetic, water)
- Exposure is dried with sterile cotton or sterile paper point
- Some clinicians feel that clot should not be allowed to form before placement of medicament
- Exposure is coated with material of choice
- Permanent restoration is placed directly over medicament or a base is placed first, depending upon permanent restoration type
- Patient is recalled periodically for evidence of signs or symptoms of irreversible pulpitis or pulpal necrosis

JUDGING CLINICAL SUCCESS AFTER DIRECT PULP-CAPPING PROCEDURE

- Patient asymptomatic
- No evidence of radiographic changes indicating pathosis

- Patient can function on tooth
- Soft tissue within normal limits
- Normal development of radicular tooth structure

Indirect Pulp-Capping Therapy

- Controversial procedure (particularly in permanent teeth)
- Defined as a treatment that purposefully prevents exposure of the pulp by allowing affected dentin to remain next to pulpal tissue that would have caused an exposure of the pulp if it were removed
- Purpose of Indirect Pulp Cap
    - Preserve vitality of the pulp
    - Prevent pulpal exposure
    - Remove infected dentin
    - Formation of reparative or tertiary dentin
    - Maintain space for permanent tooth eruption
    - Maintain support and function of primary tooth
- Usually a two-appointment procedure (controversial)
- Higher rates of success than direct pulp-capping procedure in primary teeth
- Contraindicated when signs (clinical or radiographic) and/or symptoms indicate irreversible pulpitis is present
    - Radiographic evidence of periradicular pathosis
    - Spontaneous pain from tooth
    - Sinus tract present or soft tissue swelling
    - Percussion sensitivity
    - Hemorrhage occurs during removal of caries
    - Severe and/or lingering pain from thermal tests

INDIRECT PULP-CAPPING MATERIALS

- Calcium hydroxide
- Zinc oxide
- Stannous fluoride
- IRM

JUDGING CLINICAL SUCCESS AFTER DIRECT PULP-CAPPING PROCEDURE

- Patient asymptomatic
- No evidence of radiographic changes indicating pathosis
- Patient can function on tooth
- Soft tissue within normal limits
- Normal development of radicular tooth structure

INDIRECT PULP-CAPPING TECHNIQUE

First Appointment

- Isolation with rubber dam
- Carious dentin is removed up to point that additional removal will result in pulpal exposure
- Cautious use of a round bur in the slow speed will prevent inadvertent exposure of pulp
- Excavators can also be used for removal of carious dentin
- Area should be well irrigated after removal of all infected dentin
- Dry affected dentin and cavity prep with air syringe
- Place medicament of choice over area of affected dentin
- Restoration (composite, amalgam) is placed directly over medicament
- Patient is recalled in 8-10 weeks

Second Appointment

- Isolation with rubber dam
- Permanent restoration is removed as is the medicament placed over the treated site
- Any remaining caries is removed completely
- Care must be exercised so as not to "push forcefully" into the previously affected dentin with an explorer tip as this layer may be quite thin
- A layer of calcium hydroxide or zinc oxide is placed once again over the area
- A permanent restoration is placed (composite, amalgam, stainless steel crown)
- Patient is recalled periodically for signs/symptoms of irreversible pulpitis or pulpal necrosis

C. PULPOTOMY PROCEDURES IN PRIMARY TEETH

- Indicated when no evidence of periradicular pathosis is present

- Necessity to maintain tooth in arch for space requirements, etc

- Indicated when patient symptoms indicate irreversible pulpitis
    - No radiographic evidence of periradicular pathosis
    - Spontaneous pain from tooth
    - No percussion sensitivity
    - Severe and/or lingering pain from thermal tests
    - Vitality tests are positive
    - Tooth is restorable
    - Large and/or deep carious exposure and direct pulp cap contraindicated

MEDICAMENTS / TECHNIQUES USED FOR PRIMARY TEETH PULPOTOMY

- Formocresol
    - Highly toxic even at low concentrations
    - Can be diluted 1:5 with glycerin and water as vehicle
- Calcium hydroxide
    - Bactericidal
    - Very high pH
    - May be mixed with barium sulfate (6-8:1) for increased radiopacity
- Glutaraldehyde
    - Antimicrobial
    - Usually used in concentrations ranging from 2% to 4%
    - Noncarcinogenic
    - Fixes proteins
- Ferric sulfate
    - Antibacterial
    - Astringent agent
    - Extremely caustic to tissues

- Electrosurgery
  - Eliminates introduction of chemicals/medicaments to patient
  - Rapid
  - Instant hemostasis

PULPOTOMY TECHNIQUE WITH FORMOCRESOL

- Tooth is isolated with rubber dam
- Caries is removed completely
- Pulpotomy procedure is performed with a round bur
- Explorers and other instruments (files) are not introduced into the root canal system(s)
- Hemostasis is achieved with pressure and cotton pellets or weak astringents
- Cotton pellet is first wetted in formocresol and placed directly on the exposed pulp tissue at the orifice of the canal(s)
- Formocresol pellet remains in place for 1-5 minutes and is removed
- ZOE is placed directly over pulp stump(s)
- Permanent restoration is placed

D. ROOT CANAL PROCEDURES IN PRIMARY TEETH

- Indicated when retention of primary tooth with irreversible pulpitis (with periradicular evidence of inflammation) or necrotic pulp is required
- Pulpal tissue is removed with conventional root canal therapy techniques
- Use sodium hypochlorite as an irrigant as with permanent teeth treatment
- Great caution must be exercised during cleaning and shaping, as the canals are very small, tortuous, and easily ledged and/or perforated with too large files or rotary instruments
- Must have resorbable obturation material
- Materials used for obturation of primary teeth
  - Zinc oxide-eugenol (material of choice)

- Iodoform paste-KRI paste (iodoform, camphor, p-chlorophenol, and menthol)
- Calcium hydroxide
- Vitapex
- Maisto's paste

- Gutta-percha is contraindicated, it is not resorbable
- Obturation techniques
  - Lentulo spiral
  - Jiffy tube
  - Amalgam carrier and pluggers
  - Various syringe types
- Tooth is restored in usual manner

Chapter XXI

Endodontic Surgery

ENDODONTIC SURGERY

- Choose surgery when access to the root canal system or removal of the causative agents for pulpal or periradicular disease states cannot be accomplished via nonsurgical root canal treatment

- Implies that nonsurgical treatment failed; if plausible, nonsurgical retreatment of the root canal system is indicated prior to choosing surgical entry in the majority of cases

- Some cases require surgical intervention as the primary mode of treatment

- Phases of periradicular surgical treatment

    - Patient preparation

    - Anesthesia and hemostasis

    - Soft tissue incision and reflection

    - Access through bone to root apex or defect

    - Periradicular curettage

    - Root-end resection (apicoectomy)

    - Root-end preparation (retropreparation)

    - Root-end filling (retrograde filling) and materials

    - Closure of surgical site and postsurgical considerations

A. PATIENT PREPARATION

- Preoperative NSAIDs indicated – one day

- Preoperative rinsing with 0.12% Chlorhexidine indicated – one day

- Ensure use of preoperative antibiotics if indicated for systemic problems

- If sedation required, ensure proper management of such

- Check all other medications and ensure patient assistance in returning home if necessary

- Ensure that a good radiograph, taken from a reproducible angle is available

- Ensure all consent forms are completed and signed

B. ANESTHESIA AND HEMOSTASIS

- Profound anesthesia and hemostasis essential – achieved with combination of anesthetics and vasoconstrictors

  Lidocaine with 1:100,000 epinephrine – 1.8-3.6 mL

  Lidocaine with 1:50,000 epinephrine – 1.8 mL

---

* * * * *   Clinical Note   * * * * *

These are recommended solutions, concentrations and
amounts. Nature of anesthetic solution, amounts,
and concentrations may vary depending on the
clinician, the health history of the patient,
and the nature of the surgical procedure.

C. SOFT TISSUE INCISION AND REFLECTION

- Incisions made with #11, 12 or 15 scalpel blades through the loose alveolar mucosa and attached gingiva to the bone
- Incisions made in the gingival sulcus (full mucoperiosteal tissue flap) or in the loose alveolar mucosa/attached gingiva (submarginal tissue flap)
- Full mucoperiosteal tissue flaps have no, one, or two vertical relaxing incisions to enhance tissue retraction
  - Identified as envelope, triangular, or rectangular tissue flap, respectively
- Submarginal tissue flaps – semilunar or an attached gingiva tissue flap
- Incised tissue reflected using an undermining elevation technique – supports and enhances the lifting of the periosteum with the other soft tissues
- Split-thickness tissue elevation not indicated routinely in endodontic surgical procedures
- Periosteal elevators used to lift the tissue from the bone
- Do not remove residual tissue tags attached to the bone during and after full tissue reflection
- Assist in tissue flap stabilization when repositioned
- Do not remove periodontal ligament fibers that were severed around the coronal root surface during the incision
- Enhance tissue reattachment
- Tissue held from the surgical site to enhance vision and access to the bone with a periosteal retractor

***** **Clinical Note** *****

Newer, microsurgical blades are available with different blade angles and cutting edges. Choice of these over the traditional blades at discretion of clinician, but no studies have demonstrated the enhanced efficacy of these new instruments.

D. ACCESS THROUGH THE BONE TO THE ROOT APEX OR DEFECT

- Access through the bone with rotary burs using a coolant to minimize heat generated
  - Common burs are #6 or #8 round burs
  - Have the least impact on heat generation
- Cutting done in a shaving manner (superficial osteotomy) to reduce heat and enhance visibility
- Sterile saline the preferred irrigant, followed by sterile water
- Curettes used to expose the root apex or radicular defect, if the cortical plate of bone is missing (fenestration, dehiscence)
- Remove sufficient bone to expose surgical site and to enhance performance of surgical root-end procedures (periradicular curettage, root-end resection, root-end preparation, root-end filling)

***** **Clinical Note** *****

Both high-speed and slow-speed handpieces are advocated for use during access through the bone. Copious irrigation is essential.

E. PERIRADICULAR CURETTAGE

- Effective removal of periradicular soft tissue imperative to see the root apex
- Elimination of the majority of the reactive, inflammatory tissue
- Creates environment conducive to rapid regeneration with normal tissues
- Outer portions of tissue generally reparative in nature
- Full removal of all tissue desirable, but may not be possible
- Performed with bone curettes and periodontal scalers

- Good hemostasis minimizes hemorrhage during curettage
- Effective curettage may require resection of the root end

---

* * * * * Clinical Note * * * * *

Curettes are used in a reverse or peeling manner along the lateral borders of the soft tissue and in a scooping and/or scraping manner in the depths of the lesion.

F. ROOT-END RESECTION (Apicoectomy)

- Removes irregularities in the root canal system at the root apex – natural or those created by the clinician
- Provides direct access to the canal system that could not be managed nonsurgically
- Resection done with a tapered straight fissure bur or diamond bur
- Resection usually done using a solution of sterile saline or water as an irrigation
- Expose entire root end thereby exposing all canal spaces
- Curette any soft tissues located behind the resected root end
- Resect root-end (3-5 mm) at a 0-45° angle to the buccal depending on surgical visibility and need to gain access to the entire root face for proper management
- Paint resected surface with 1% methylene blue and examine for fractures or aberrant canals

G. ROOT-END PREPARATION (Retropreparation)

- Performed to seal the apical opening(s) of the root canal system
- Performed with a bur or ultrasonic tip that is bent to gain access to the resected root face
- May not be necessary in cases when the canal is cleaned, shaped, and obturated immediately prior to or during the surgical procedure
- Isolate surgical area with local hemostatic agents (collagen-based or ferric sulfate-based), if necessary

- Depth of preparation should be at least 3-4 mm, but not limited to such

- Shape of preparation must encompass all exposed canal space

- If using bur preparation, microburs essential as is a miniature handpiece for access to the confined surgical area

- If using an ultrasonic preparation technique, minimize time, energy, and pressure during cutting to lessen chance for possible root fractures

- Ultrasonic technique should have internal irrigation for debris removal and temperature reduction during preparation

- Prepare with ultrasonic or bur in the long axis of the root to prevent root perforations

- Consider rinsing root-end cavity with liquid EDTA (ethylenediaminetetraacetic acid) or 10% citric acid prior to placement of a restoration to remove smear layer

- Rinse with sterile water and dry with paper points

- Use a micromirror or small dental mirror to see root-end cavity if necessary

- Preparation may be cut under microscopic visualization, if available

H. ROOT-END FILLING – MATERIALS

- Once apical cavity prepared, place restorative material
  - Isolation from fluids is necessary
  - Cavity must be dry

- Material compacted and surface finished – avoid flash on resected root face

- Remove material particles from the surgical site prior to surgical closure

- Remove hemostatic agents unless used to enhance bone formation in the surgical site

- **Contemporary root-end fillings include:**
  - Super EBA (o-ethoxybenzoic acid)
  - IRM (zinc oxide-eugenol base)
  - MTA (mineral trioxide aggregate)

---

* * * * * **Clinical Note** * * * * *

Amalgam has fallen into disfavor by some
as a root-end filling material.

I. CLOSURE OF THE SURGICAL SITE – POSTSURGICAL CONSIDERATIONS

- Sutures used routinely to close the surgical site

- 3-0, 4-0, 5-0 silk or gut sutures, or a combination thereof, may be used to reattach the tissue

- Complete closure should be obtained

- Expose final radiograph, taken at same angle as initial film

- After suturing, compression with moist gauze for 3-5 minutes

- Use of ibuprofen for pain management

- Place ice or cold compresses externally on the surgical site for 15-20 minutes followed by removal for 15-20 minutes and replaced for 15-20, etc, during the day of the surgery is recommended strongly, if possible

- Use hot saline rinses for the day following the surgery and until the sutures are removed

- Chlorhexidine may be used for 3-5 days

---

* * * * * Clinical Note * * * * *

The routine administration of antibiotics following surgery has no scientific basis and is not recommended.

J. SURGICAL ROOT OR TOOTH RESECTIONS

- Removal of a root or roots, along with a portion of the tooth crown, may be indicated

  INDICATIONS
  - Extensive periodontal disease
  - Inoperable endodontically
  - Unmanageable defect
  - Anatomically misplaced

- Tooth may require the removal of a root – root resection (amputation) or the tooth may be sectioned into two segments – tooth resection (hemisection) or in some cases three segments (trisection)

- In case of a root resection, crown may remain intact, or a segment of the crown may be removed

ROOT RESECTION

- Careful and thorough treatment planning when choosing as treatment modality

- Performed primarily on maxillary or mandibular molars

- Roots must be separated

- Furcation must be located in a coronal position – preferably above the bony crest

- Probings must delineate position of the bone circumferentially around the root to be resected

- Use both straight (Michigan type) and curved (Nabors) probes

- Full mucoperiosteal surgical tissue flaps – when the root is not exposed from periodontal disease

- Use long or extra long, tapered, thin fissure or diamond burs for resection

- Resection must be smooth, blending into the furcation and avoiding the retained root

- Make cuts favoring the retained root – surfaces and margins finished after root segment removal

- Good surgical vision and multiple-angled radiographs necessary to envision the three-dimensional aspects of the cut tooth surface

- Tooth usually requires full coronal coverage restoration

- Alter occlusion to reduce the functional forces placed on the crown over resected area

TOOTH RESECTION

- Careful and thorough treatment planning when choosing as treatment modality

- Performed on maxillary or mandibular molars

- Hemisection performed on mandibular molars only

- Roots must be separated – many mandibular second molars have fused roots

- Furcation must be located in a coronal position – preferably above the bony crest

- Probings must delineate position of bone circumferentially around the root to be resected

- Use both straight (Michigan type) and curved (Nabors) probes

- Full mucoperiosteal surgical tissue flaps – when the root is not exposed from periodontal disease

- Necessitates reflection of both buccal and lingual tissue

- Use long or extra long, tapered, thin fissure or diamond burs for resection

- Resection must be smooth, blending into the furcation and avoiding the retained root

- Mandibular molars – the buccal and lingual developmental grooves can be used as a guide for the bur cut

- Make cuts favoring the retained root – surfaces and margins finished after root segment removal

- Good surgical vision and multiple-angled radiographs necessary to envision the three-dimensional aspects of the cut tooth surface

- Tooth usually requires full coronal coverage restoration

- Alter occlusion to reduce the functional forces placed on the crown over resected area

- If both segments are retained, roots must be separated sufficiently and the cut must be done to ensure that neither root has been gouged or damaged

- Orthodontic root movement can follow the resection procedure to separate the roots, if necessary

---

* * * * * Clinical Note * * * * *

The biggest causes of failure with this treatment procedure are 1) lack of proper treatment planning; 2) failure to adjust the occlusion and redistribute the occlusal forces; 3) resections that leave deep, unrestorable, and nonmaintainable tooth margins; and; 4) errors in the resection technique that either result in the gouging of the adjacent roots or the presence of irregular root spurs from an incomplete resection.

K. SURGICAL REPAIR OF PERFORATIONS

- Depends on access to defect
- Relationship of perforation to crestal bone and epithelial attachment critical

LOCATION OF PERFORATION

- Apical-third perforations pose little problem – removed during resection
- Mid-root perforations difficult because of accessibility and radiographic interpretation
- Must use buccal object rule to locate accurately
- Must gain surgical access without compromising root and bone
- If root canal filled, use simple preparation and seal with MTA or other root-end filling materials (see above)
- If due to post, grinding of post may be difficult
- If post not cemented, repair perforation and reduce post length
- Perforation on mesial or distal surface difficult to gain access
- Lingual perforations almost impossible to repair surgically – must rethink and consider repair through the canal
- Always possible to create periodontal defects with mid-root surgical repairs – especially in the furcation
- May require the concomitant placement of a guided tissue membrane or bone substitute graft
- Coronal root perforations challenging if at crest or slightly below
- Above bony crest – restore directly or use small tissue flap to expose
- Below bony crest – may require concomitant crown lengthening
- Restore with materials compatible with environment of oral cavity (eg, bonded composites, copolymers, etc); do not use MTA
- Could also consider orthodontic or surgical root extrusion to elevate defect
- Treatment plan to prevent or manage any periodontal defects

FREQUENTLY ASKED QUESTIONS (FAQs)

1. *Is amalgam still a viable choice as a root-end filling material?*

   The use of amalgam as a root-end filling material is not advocated in contemporary endodontic surgery. However, an exception to this guideline would be that, if used, it should be placed in moisture-controlled environment along with an acceptable bonding agent.

2. *Is the use of the "semilunar" tissue flap acceptable in contemporary endodontic surgery?*

   Yes — the semilunar tissue flap design is quite acceptable, but its choice as the primary method of soft tissue entry has been reduced in popularity. Some of the reasons for this are empirical. The semilunar tissue flap should be considered in the anterior maxilla when specific parameters dictate.

3. *How much of the root apex should be resected during apical surgery?*

   Resection is done for a myriad of reasons. However, some of the more important reasons that will dictate the amount of resection are 1) apical resorption; 2) dentist created apical defects; 3) unmanaged canal space; and 4) severe anatomical irregularities. Generally 3-5 mm of resection is sufficient.

4. *I heard that the use of silk sutures is contraindicated because of infections that occur around this material – is this true?*

   Any suture material that serves as a trap for food debris and bacteria can cause localized inflammation and possible infection. Silk sutures are quite acceptable and, as with any sutured wound regardless of the suture material, they should be kept clean, preferably with chlorhexidine rinses.

5. *Is the use of citric acid indicated on the root apex before tissue replacement and suturing?*

   Citric acid (50%) has been shown, following application on the resected root ends of dogs, to enhance possibly cemental deposition. There are other reports that indicate that this is not necessary to achieve this level of tissue regeneration in the human. If used, a 10% solution is recommended, lightly burnishing the root end for approximately 1 minute.

6. *Are antibiotics indicated routinely after endodontic surgery?*

The routine use of antibiotics subsequent to endodontic surgery is not indicated. There are some circumstances that will dictate the use of antibiotics however, such as systemic conditions that require premedication, entry into the sinus cavity, and a history of chronic sinus infections. Each case has to be evaluated on its own merit.

APPENDIX TABLE OF CONTENTS

ABBREVIATIONS, ACRONYMS, AND SYMBOLS

Abbreviation	Meaning
aa, aā	of each
AA	Alcoholics Anonymous
ac	before meals or food
ad	to, up to
a.d.	right ear
ADHD	attention-deficit/hyperactivity disorder
ADLs	activities of daily living
ad lib	at pleasure
AIMS	Abnormal Involuntary Movement Scale
a.l.	left ear
AM	morning
amp	ampul
amt	amount
aq	water
aq. dest.	distilled water
a.s.	left ear
ASAP	as soon as possible
a.u.	each ear
AUC	area under the curve
BDI	Beck Depression Inventory
bid	twice daily
bm	bowel movement
bp	blood pressure
BPRS	Brief Psychiatric Rating Scale
BSA	body surface area
c̱	a gallon
c	with
cal	calorie
cap	capsule
CBT	cognitive behavioral therapy
cc	cubic centimeter
CGI	Clinical Global Impression
cm	centimeter
CIV	continuous I.V. infusion
comp	compound
cont	continue
CT	computed tomography
d	day
d/c	discontinue
dil	dilute
disp	dispense

Abbreviation	Meaning
div	divide
DSM-IV	Diagnostic and Statistical Manual
DTs	delirium tremens
dtd	give of such a dose
ECT	electroconvulsive therapy
EEG	electroencephalogram
elix, el	elixir
emp	as directed
EPS	extrapyramidal side effects
et	and
ex aq	in water
f, ft	make, let be made
FDA	Food and Drug Administration
g	gram
GA	Gamblers Anonymous
GAD	generalized anxiety disorder
GAF	Global Assessment of Functioning Scale
GABA	gamma-aminobutyric acid
GITS	gastrointestinal therapeutic system
gr	grain
gtt	a drop
h	hour
HAM-A	Hamilton Anxiety Scale
HAM-D	Hamilton Depression Scale
hs	at bedtime
I.M.	intramuscular
IU	international unit
I.V.	intravenous
kcal	kilocalorie
kg	kilogram
KIU	kallikrein inhibitor unit
L	liter
LAMM	L-α-acetyl methadol
liq	a liquor, solution
M.	mix
MADRS	Montgomery Asbery Depression Rating Scale
MAOIs	monamine oxidase inhibitors
mcg	microgram
MDEA	3,4-methylene-dioxy amphetamine
m. dict	as directed
MDMA	3,4-methylene-dioxy methamphetamine
mEq	milliequivalent
mg	milligram
mixt	a mixture

Abbreviation	Meaning
mL	milliliter
mm	millimeter
MMSE	Mini-Mental State Examination
MPPP	l-methyl-4-proprionoxy-4-phenyl pyridine
MR	mental retardation
MRI	magnetic resonance imaging
NF	National Formulary
NMS	neuroleptic malignant syndrome
no.	number
noc	in the night
non rep	do not repeat, no refills
NPO	nothing by mouth
O, Oct	a pint
OCD	obsessive-compulsive disorder
o.d.	right eye
o.l.	left eye
o.s.	left eye
o.u.	each eye
PANSS	Positive and Negative Symptom Scale
pc, post cib	after meals
PCP	phencyclidine
per	through or by
PM	afternoon or evening
P.O.	by mouth
P.R.	rectally
prn	as needed
PTSD	post-traumatic stress disorder
pulv	a powder
q	every
qad	every other day
qd	every day
qh	every hour
qid	four times a day
qod	every other day
qs	a sufficient quantity
qs ad	a sufficient quantity to make
qty	quantity
qv	as much as you wish
REM	rapid eye movement
Rx	take, a recipe
rep	let it be repeated
s	without
sa	according to art
sat	saturated

Abbreviation	Meaning
S.C.	subcutaneous
sig	label, or let it be printed
sol	solution
solv	dissolve
ss	one-half
sos	if there is need
SSRIs	selective serotonin reuptake inhibitors
stat	at once, immediately
supp	suppository
syr	syrup
tab	tablet
tal	such
TCA	tricyclic antidepressant
TD	tardive dyskinesia
tid	three times a day
tr, tinct	tincture
trit	triturate
tsp	teaspoonful
ULN	upper limits of normal
ung	ointment
USAN	United States Adopted Names
USP	United States Pharmacopeia
u.d., ut dict	as directed
v.o.	verbal order
w.a.	while awake
x3	3 times
x4	4 times
YBOC	Yale Brown Obsessive-Compulsive Scale
YMRS	Young Mania Rating Scale

APOTHECARY / METRIC EQUIVALENTS

Approximate Liquid Measures

Basic equivalent: 1 fluid ounce = 30 mL

Examples:

1 gallon	3800 mL	1 gallon	128 fluid ounces
1 quart	960 mL	1 quart	32 fluid ounces
1 pint	480 mL	1 pint	16 fluid ounces
8 fluid oz	240 mL	15 minims	1 mL
4 fluid oz	120 mL	10 minims	0.6 mL

Approximate Household Equivalents

1 teaspoonful	5 mL	1 tablespoonful	15 mL

Weights

Basic equivalents:

1 oz	30 g	15 gr	1 g

Examples:

4 oz	120 g	1 gr	60 mg
2 oz	60 g	1/100 gr	600 mcg
10 gr	600 mg	1/150 gr	400 mcg
7½ gr	500 mg	1/200 gr	300 mcg
16 oz	1 lb		

Metric Conversions

Basic equivalents:

1 g	1000 mg	1 mg	1000 mcg

Examples:

5 g	5000 mg	5 mg	5000 mcg
0.5 g	500 mg	0.5 g	500 mcg
0.05 g	50 mg	0.05 mg	50 mcg

Exact Equivalents

1 g	=	15.43 gr
1 mL	=	16.23 minims
1 minim	=	0.06 mL
1 gr	=	64.8 mg
1 pint (pt)	=	473.2 mL
1 oz	=	28.35 g
1 lb	=	453.6 g
1 kg	=	2.2 lbs
1 qt	=	946.4 mL

0.1 mg	=	1/600 gr
0.12 mg	=	1/500 gr
0.15 mg	=	1/400 gr
0.2 mg	=	1/300 gr
0.3 mg	=	1/200 gr
0.4 mg	=	1/150 gr
0.5 mg	=	1/120 gr
0.6 mg	=	1/100 gr
0.8 mg	=	1/80 gr
1 mg	=	1/65 gr

Solids*

1/4 grain	=	15 mg
1/2 grain	=	30 mg
1 grain	=	60 mg
1 1/2 grains	=	90 mg
5 grains	=	300 mg
10 grains	=	600 mg

*Use exact equivalents for compounding and calculations requiring a high degree of accuracy.

AVERAGE WEIGHTS AND SURFACE AREAS

Average Weight and Surface Area of Preterm Infants, Term Infants, and Children

Age	Average Weight (kg)*	Approximate Surface Area (m²)
Weeks Gestation		
26	0.9-1	0.1
30	1.3-1.5	0.12
32	1.6-2	0.15
38	2.9-3	0.2
40 (term infant at birth)	3.1-4	0.25
Months		
3	5	0.29
6	7	0.38
9	8	0.42
Year		
1	10	0.49
2	12	0.55
3	15	0.64
4	17	0.74
5	18	0.76
6	20	0.82
7	23	0.90
8	25	0.95
9	28	1.06
10	33	1.18
11	35	1.23
12	40	1.34
Adults	70	1.73

*Weights from age 3 months and older are rounded off to the nearest kilogram.

BODY SURFACE AREA OF ADULTS AND CHILDREN

Calculating Body Surface Area in Children

In a child of average size, find weight and corresponding surface area on the boxed scale to the left; or, use the nomogram to the right. Lay a straightedge on the correct height and weight points for the child, then read the intersecting point on the surface area scale.

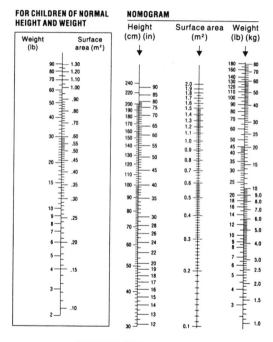

FOR CHILDREN OF NORMAL HEIGHT AND WEIGHT

NOMOGRAM

BODY SURFACE AREA FORMULA
(Adult and Pediatric)

$$BSA\ (m^2) = \sqrt{\frac{Ht\ (in)\ x\ Wt\ (lb)}{3131}} \quad \text{or, in metric:} \quad BSA\ (m^2) = \sqrt{\frac{Ht\ (cm)\ x\ Wt\ (kg)}{3600}}$$

References

Lam TK and Leung DT, "More on Simplified Calculation of Body Surface Area," *N Engl J Med*, 1988, 318(17):1130 (Letter).
Mosteller RD, "Simplified Calculation of Body Surface Area", *N Engl J Med*, 1987, 317(17):1098 (Letter).

IDEAL BODY WEIGHT CALCULATION

Adults (18 years and older) (IBW is in kg)

IBW (male) = 50 + (2.3 x height in inches over 5 feet)

IBW (female) = 45.5 + (2.3 x height in inches over 5 feet)

Children (IBW is in kg; height is in cm)

a. 1-18 years

$$IBW = \frac{(height^2 \times 1.65)}{1000}$$

b. 5 feet and taller

IBW (male) = 39 + (2.27 x height in inches over 5 feet)

IBW (female) = 42.2 + (2.27 x height in inches over 5 feet)

MILLIEQUIVALENT AND MILLIMOLE CALCULATIONS & CONVERSIONS

DEFINITIONS & CALCULATIONS

Definitions

mole	=	gram molecular weight of a substance (aka molar weight)
millimole (mM)	=	milligram molecular weight of a substance (a millimole is 1/1000 of a mole)
equivalent weight	=	gram weight of a substance which will combine with or replace one gram (one mole) of hydrogen; an equivalent weight can be determined by dividing the molar weight of a substance by its ionic valence
milliequivalent (mEq)	=	milligram weight of a substance which will combine with or replace one milligram (one millimole) of hydrogen (a milliequivalent is 1/1000 of an equivalent)

Calculations

moles	=	$\dfrac{\text{weight of a substance (grams)}}{\text{molecular weight of that substance (grams)}}$
millimoles	=	$\dfrac{\text{weight of a substance (milligrams)}}{\text{molecular weight of that substance (milligrams)}}$
equivalents	=	moles x valence of ion
milliequivalents	=	millimoles x valence of ion
moles	=	$\dfrac{\text{equivalents}}{\text{valence of ion}}$
millimoles	=	$\dfrac{\text{milliequivalents}}{\text{valence of ion}}$
millimoles	=	moles x 1000
milliequivalents	=	equivalents x 1000

Note: Use of equivalents and milliequivalents is valid only for those substances which have fixed ionic valences (eg, sodium, potassium, calcium, chlorine, magnesium bromine, etc). For substances with variable ionic valences (eg, phosphorous), a reliable equivalent value cannot be determined. In these instances, one should calculate millimoles (which are fixed and reliable) rather than milliequivalents.

MILLIEQUIVALENT CONVERSIONS

To convert mg/100 mL to mEq/L the following formula may be used:

$$\frac{(mg/100\ mL) \times 10 \times valence}{atomic\ weight} = mEq/L$$

To convert mEq/L to mg/100 mL the following formula may be used:

$$\frac{(mEq/L) \times atomic\ weight}{10 \times valence} = mg/100\ mL$$

To convert mEq/L to volume of percent of a gas the following formula may be used:

$$\frac{(mEq/L) \times 22.4}{10} = volume\ percent$$

Valences and Atomic Weights of Selected Ions

Substance	Electrolyte	Valence	Molecular Wt
Calcium	Ca^{++}	2	40
Chloride	Cl^-	1	35.5
Magnesium	Mg^{++}	2	24
Phosphate	HPO_4^{--} (80%)	1.8	96*
pH = 7.4	$H_2PO_4^-$ (20%)	1.8	96*
Potassium	K^+	1	39
Sodium	Na^+	1	23
Sulfate	SO_4^{--}	2	96*

*The molecular weight of phosphorus only is 31, and sulfur only is 32.

Approximate Milliequivalents — Weights of Selected Ions

Salt	mEq/g Salt	Mg Salt/mEq
Calcium carbonate ($CaCO_3$)	20	50
Calcium chloride ($CaCl_2 \bullet 2H_2O$)	14	73
Calcium gluconate (Ca gluconate$_2 \bullet 1H_2O$)	4	224
Calcium lactate (Ca lactate$_2 \bullet 5H_2O$)	6	154
Magnesium sulfate ($MgSO_4$)	16	60
Magnesium sulfate ($MgSO_4 \bullet 7H_2O$)	8	123
Potassium acetate (K acetate)	10	98
Potassium chloride (KCl)	13	75
Potassium citrate (K_3 citrate $\bullet 1H_2O$)	9	108
Potassium iodide (KI)	6	166
Sodium bicarbonate ($NaHCO_3$)	12	84
Sodium chloride (NaCl)	17	58
Sodium citrate (Na_3 citrate $\bullet 2H_2O$)	10	98
Sodium iodine (NaI)	7	150
Sodium lactate (Na lactate)	9	112

CORRECTED SODIUM

Corrected Na^+ = measured Na^+ + [1.5 x (glucose − 150 divided by 100)]

Note: Do not correct for glucose <150.

WATER DEFICIT

Water deficit = 0.6 x body weight [1 − (140 divided by Na^+)]

Note: Body weight is estimated weight in kg when fully hydrated; **Na^+** is serum or plasma sodium. Use corrected Na^+ if necessary. Consult medical references for recommendations for replacement of deficit.

TOTAL SERUM CALCIUM CORRECTED FOR ALBUMIN LEVEL

[(Normal albumin − patient's albumin) x 0.8] + patient's measured total calcium

ACID-BASE ASSESSMENT

Henderson-Hasselbalch Equation

$$pH = 6.1 + \log (HCO_3^- / (0.03) (pCO_2))$$

Alveolar Gas Equation

PIO_2	=	FiO_2 x (total atmospheric pressure − vapor pressure of H_2O at 37°C)
	=	FiO_2 x (760 mm Hg − 47 mm Hg)
PAO_2	=	PIO_2 − $PACO_2$ / R

Alveolar/arterial oxygen gradient = PAO_2 − PaO_2

Normal ranges:

Children	15-20 mm Hg
Adults	20-25 mm Hg

where:

PIO_2	=	Oxygen partial pressure of inspired gas (mm Hg) (150 mm Hg in room air at sea level)
FiO_2	=	Fractional pressure of oxygen in inspired gas (0.21 in room air)
PAO_2	=	Alveolar oxygen partial pressure
$PACO_2$	=	Alveolar carbon dioxide partial pressure
PaO_2	=	Arterial oxygen partial pressure
R	=	Respiratory exchange quotient (typically 0.8, increases with high carbohydrate diet, decreases with high fat diet)

Acid-Base Disorders

Acute metabolic acidosis (<12 h duration):

$$PaCO_2 \text{ expected} \approx 1.5 \, (HCO_3^-) + 8 \pm 2$$

or

expected change in pCO = (1-1.5) x change in HCO_3^-

Acute metabolic alkalosis (<12 h duration):

expected change in pCO_2 = (0.5-1) x change in HCO_3^-

Acute respiratory acidosis (<6 h duration):

expected change in HCO_3^- = 0.1 x pCO_2

Acute respiratory acidosis (>6 h duration):

expected change in HCO_3^- = 0.4 x change in pCO_2

Acute respiratory alkalosis (<6 h duration):

expected change in HCO_3^- = 0.2 x change in pCO_2

Acute respiratory alkalosis (>6 h duration):

expected change in HCO_3^- = 0.5 x change in pCO_2

ACID-BASE EQUATION

H^+ (in mEq/L) = (24 x $PaCO_2$) divided by HCO_3^-

Aa GRADIENT

Aa gradient $[(713)(FiO_2 - (PaCO_2 \text{ divided by } 0.8))] - PaO_2$

Aa gradient	=	alveolar-arterial oxygen gradient
FiO_2	=	inspired oxygen (expressed as a fraction)
$PaCO_2$	=	arterial partial pressure carbon dioxide (mm Hg)
PaO_2	=	arterial partial pressure oxygen (mm Hg)

OSMOLALITY

Definition: The summed concentrations of all osmotically active solute particles.

Predicted serum osmolality =
   2 Na^+ + glucose (mg/dL) / 18 + BUN (mg/dL) / 2.8

The normal range of serum osmolality is 285-295 mOsm/L.

266

Differential diagnosis of increased serum osmolal gap (>10 mOsm/L)

Medications and toxins
Alcohols (ethanol, methanol, isopropanol, glycerol, ethylene
glycol)
Mannitol
Paraldehyde

Calculated Osm

Osmolal gap = measured Osm − calculated Osm

0 to +10: Normal
>10: Abnormal
<0: Probable lab or calculation error

BICARBONATE DEFICIT

HCO_3^- deficit = (0.4 x wt in kg) x (HCO_3^- desired − HCO_3^- measured)

Note: In clinical practice, the calculated quantity may differ markedly from
the actual amount of bicarbonate needed or that which may be safely
administered.

ANION GAP

Definition: The difference in concentration between unmeasured cation
and anion equivalents in serum.

Anion gap = Na^+ − Cl^- − HCO_3^-
(The normal anion gap is 10-14 mEq/L)

Differential Diagnosis of Increased Anion Gap Acidosis

Organic anions

Lactate (sepsis, hypovolemia, seizures, large tumor burden)
Pyruvate
Uremia
Ketoacidosis (β-hydroxybutyrate and acetoacetate)
Amino acids and their metabolites
Other organic acids

Inorganic anions

Hyperphosphatemia
Sulfates
Nitrates

Differential Diagnosis of Decreased Anion Gap

Organic cations

    Hypergammaglobulinemia

Inorganic cations

    Hyperkalemia
    Hypercalcemia
    Hypermagnesemia

Medications and toxins

    Lithium

Hypoalbuminemia

RETICULOCYTE INDEX

(% retic divided by 2) x (patient's Hct divided by normal Hct) or (% retic divided by 2) x (patient's Hgb divided by normal Hgb)

Normal index: 1.0
Good marrow response: 2.0-6.0

PEDIATRIC DOSAGE ESTIMATIONS

Dosage Estimations Based on Weight:

Augsberger's rule:

$$\frac{(1.5 \times \text{weight in kg} + 10)}{\% \text{ of adult dose}} = \text{child's approximate dose}$$

Clark's rule:

$$\frac{\text{weight (in pounds)}}{150} \times \text{adult dose} = \text{child's approximate dose}$$

Dosage Estimations Based on Age:

Augsberger's rule:

$$\frac{(4 \times \text{age in years} + 20)}{\% \text{ of adult dose}} = \text{child's approximate dose}$$

Bastedo's rule:

$$\frac{\text{age in years} + 3}{30} \times \text{adult dose} = \text{child's approximate dose}$$

Cowling's rule:

$$\frac{\text{age at next birthday (in years)}}{24} \times \text{adult dose} = \text{child's approximate dose}$$

Dilling's rule:

$$\frac{\text{age (in years)}}{20} \times \text{adult dose} = \text{child's approximate dose}$$

Fried's rule for infants (younger than 1 year):

$$\frac{\text{age (in months)}}{150} \times \text{adult dose} = \text{infant's approximate dose}$$

Young's rule:

$$\frac{\text{age (in years)}}{\text{age} + 12} \times \text{adult dose} = \text{child's approximate dose}$$

POUNDS / KILOGRAMS CONVERSION

1 pound = 0.45359 kilograms
1 kilogram = 2.2 pounds

lb =	kg	lb =	kg	lb =	kg
1	0.45	70	31.75	140	63.50
5	2.27	75	34.02	145	65.77
10	4.54	80	36.29	150	68.04
15	6.80	85	38.56	155	70.31
20	9.07	90	40.82	160	72.58
25	11.34	95	43.09	165	74.84
30	13.61	100	45.36	170	77.11
35	15.88	105	47.63	175	79.38
40	18.14	110	49.90	180	81.65
45	20.41	115	52.16	185	83.92
50	22.68	120	54.43	190	86.18
55	24.95	125	56.70	195	88.45
60	27.22	130	58.91	200	90.72
65	29.48	135	61.24		

TEMPERATURE CONVERSION

Celsius to Fahrenheit = (°C x 9/5) + 32 = °F
Fahrenheit to Celsius = (°F − 32) x 5/9 = °C

°C =	°F	°C =	°F	°C =	°F
100.0	212.0	39.0	102.2	36.8	98.2
50.0	122.0	38.8	101.8	36.6	97.9
41.0	105.8	38.6	101.5	36.4	97.5
40.8	105.4	38.4	101.1	36.2	97.2
40.6	105.1	38.2	100.8	36.0	96.8
40.4	104.7	38.0	100.4	35.8	96.4
40.2	104.4	37.8	100.1	35.6	96.1
40.0	104.0	37.6	99.7	35.4	95.7
39.8	103.6	37.4	99.3	35.2	95.4
39.6	103.3	37.2	99.0	35.0	95.0
39.4	102.9	37.0	98.6	0	32.0
39.2	102.6				

REFERENCE VALUES FOR ADULTS

Automated Chemistry (CHEMISTRY A)

Test	Values	Remarks
SERUM PLASMA		
Acetone	Negative	
Albumin	3.2-5 g/dL	
Alcohol, ethyl	Negative	
Aldolase	1.2-7.6 IU/L	
Ammonia	20-70 mcg/dL	Specimen to be placed on ice as soon as collected
Amylase	30-110 units/L	
Bilirubin, direct	0-0.3 mg/dL	
Bilirubin, total	0.1-1.2 mg/dL	
Calcium	8.6-10.3 mg/dL	
Calcium, ionized	2.24-2.46 mEq/L	
Chloride	95-108 mEq/L	
Cholesterol, total	≤220 mg/dL	Fasted blood required – normal value affected by dietary habits This reference range is for a general adult population
HDL cholesterol	40-60 mg/dL	Fasted blood required – normal value affected by dietary habits
LDL cholesterol	65-170 mg/dL	LDLC calculated by Friewald formula... which has certain inaccuracies and is invalid at trig levels >300 mg/dL
CO_2	23-30 mEq/L	
Creatine kinase (CK) isoenzymes		
CK-BB	0%	
CK-MB (cardiac)	0%-3.9%	
CK-MM (muscle)	96%-100%	
CK-MB levels must be both ≥4% and 10 IU/L to meet diagnostic criteria for CK-MB positive result consistent with myocardial injury.		
Creatine phosphokinase (CPK)	8-150 IU/L	
Creatinine	0.5-1.4 mg/dL	
Ferritin	13-300 ng/mL	
Folate	3.6-20 ng/dL	

Automated Chemistry (CHEMISTRY A) *(continued)*

Test	Values	Remarks
GGT (gamma-glutamyltranspeptidase)		
male	11-63 IU/L	
female	8-35 IU/L	
GLDH	To be determined	
Glucose (2-h postprandial)	Up to 140 mg/dL	
Glucose, fasting	60-110 mg/dL	
Glucose, nonfasting (2-h postprandial)	60-140 mg/dL	
Hemoglobin A$_{1c}$	8	
Hemoglobin, plasma free	<2.5 mg/100 mL	
Hemoglobin, total glycosylated (Hb A$_1$)	4%-8%	
Iron	65-150 mcg/dL	
Iron binding capacity, total (TIBC)	250-420 mcg/dL	
Lactic acid	0.7-2.1 mEq/L	Specimen to be kept on ice and sent to lab as soon as possible
Lactate dehydrogenase (LDH)	56-194 IU/L	
Lactate dehydrogenase (LDH) isoenzymes		
LD$_1$	20%-34%	
LD$_2$	29%-41%	
LD$_3$	15%-25%	
LD$_4$	1%-12%	
LD$_5$	1%-15%	
Flipped LD$_1$/LD$_2$ ratios (>1 may be consistent with myocardial injury) particularly when considered in combination with a recent CK-MB positive result		
Lipase	23-208 units/L	
Magnesium	1.6-2.5 mg/dL	Increased by slight hemolysis
Osmolality	289-308 mOsm/kg	
Phosphatase, alkaline		
adults 25-60 y	33-131 IU/L	
adults 61 y or older	51-153 IU/L	
infancy-adolescence	Values range up to 3-5 times higher than adults	
Phosphate, inorganic	2.8-4.2 mg/dL	
Potassium	3.5-5.2 mEq/L	Increased by slight hemolysis
Prealbumin	>15 mg/dL	
Protein, total	6.5-7.9 g/dL	

Automated Chemistry (CHEMISTRY A) *(continued)*

Test	Values	Remarks
SGOT (AST)	<35 IU/L (20-48)	
SGPT (ALT) (10-35)	<35 IU/L	
Sodium	134-149 mEq/L	
Transferrin	>200 mg/dL	
Triglycerides	45-155 mg/dL	Fasted blood required
Urea nitrogen (BUN)	7-20 mg/dL	
Uric acid		
male	2.0-8.0 mg/dL	
female	2.0-7.5 mg/dL	

CEREBROSPINAL FLUID

Test	Values	Remarks
Glucose	50-70 mg/dL	
Protein		
adults and children	15-45 mg/dL	CSF obtained by lumbar puncture
newborn infants	60-90 mg/dL	

On CSF obtained by cisternal puncture: About 25 mg/dL

On CSF obtained by ventricular puncture: About 10 mg/dL

Note: Bloody specimen gives erroneously high value due to contamination with blood proteins

URINE

(24-hour specimen is required for all these tests unless specified)

Test	Values	Remarks
Amylase	32-641 units/L	The value is in units/L and **not** calculated for total volume
Amylase, fluid (random samples)		Interpretation of value left for physician, depends on the nature of fluid
Calcium	Depends upon dietary intake	
Creatine		
male	150 mg/24 h	Higher value on children and during pregnancy
female	250 mg/24 h	
Creatinine	1000-2000 mg/24 h	
Creatinine clearance (endogenous)		
male	85-125 mL/min	A blood sample must accompany urine specimen
female	75-115 mL/min	
Glucose	1 g/24 h	

Automated Chemistry (CHEMISTRY A) *(continued)*

Test	Values	Remarks
5-hydroxyindoleacetic acid	2-8 mg/24 h	
Iron	0.15 mg/24 h	Acid washed container required
Magnesium	146-209 mg/24 h	
Osmolality	500-800 mOsm/kg	With normal fluid intake
Oxalate	10-40 mg/24 h	
Phosphate	400-1300 mg/24 h	
Potassium	25-120 mEq/24 h	Varies with diet; the interpretation of urine electrolytes and osmolality should be left for the physician
Sodium	40-220 mEq/24 h	
Porphobilinogen, qualitative	Negative	
Porphyrins, qualitative	Negative	
Proteins	0.05-0.1 g/24 h	
Salicylate	Negative	
Urea clearance	60-95 mL/min	A blood sample must accompany specimen
Urea N	10-40 g/24 h	Dependent on protein intake
Uric acid	250-750 mg/24 h	Dependent on diet and therapy
Urobilinogen	0.5-3.5 mg/24 h	For qualitative determination on random urine, send sample to urinalysis section in Hematology Lab
Xylose absorption test		
children	16%-33% of ingested xylose	
adults	>4 g in 5 h	
FECES		
Fat, 3-day collection	<5 g/d	Value depends on fat intake of 100 g/d for 3 days preceding and during collection
GASTRIC ACIDITY		
Acidity, total, 12 h	10-60 mEq/L	Titrated at pH 7

BLOOD GASES

	Arterial	Capillary	Venous
pH	7.35-7.45	7.35-7.45	7.32-7.42
pCO_2 (mm Hg)	35-45	35-45	38-52
pO_2 (mm Hg)	70-100	60-80	24-48
HCO_3 (mEq/L)	19-25	19-25	19-25
TCO_2 (mEq/L)	19-29	19-29	23-33
O_2 saturation (%)	90-95	90-95	40-70
Base excess (mEq/L)	-5 to +5	-5 to +5	-5 to +5

HEMATOLOGY

Complete Blood Count

Age	Hgb (g/dL)	Hct (%)	RBC (mill/mm³)	RDW
0-3 d	15.0-20.0	45-61	4.0-5.9	<18
1-2 wk	12.5-18.5	39-57	3.6-5.5	<17
1-6 mo	10.0-13.0	29-42	3.1-4.3	<16.5
7 mo to 2 y	10.5-13.0	33-38	3.7-4.9	<16
2-5 y	11.5-13.0	34-39	3.9-5.0	<15
5-8 y	11.5-14.5	35-42	4.0-4.9	<15
13-18 y	12.0-15.2	36-47	4.5-5.1	<14.5
Adult male	13.5-16.5	41-50	4.5-5.5	<14.5
Adult female	12.0-15.0	36-44	4.0-4.9	<14.5

Age	MCV (fL)	MCH (pg)	MCHC (%)	Plts (x 10³/mm³)
0-3 d	95-115	31-37	29-37	250-450
1-2 wk	86-110	28-36	28-38	250-450
1-6 mo	74-96	25-35	30-36	300-700
7 mo to 2 y	70-84	23-30	31-37	250-600
2-5 y	75-87	24-30	31-37	250-550
5-8 y	77-95	25-33	31-37	250-550
13-18 y	78-96	25-35	31-37	150-450
Adult male	80-100	26-34	31-37	150-450
Adult female	80-100	26-34	31-37	150-450

WBC and Diff

Age	WBC (x 10³/mm³)	Segs	Bands	Lymphs	Monos
0-3 d	9.0-35.0	32-62	10-18	19-29	5-7
1-2 wk	5.0-20.0	14-34	6-14	36-45	6-10
1-6 mo	6.0-17.5	13-33	4-12	41-71	4-7
7 mo to 2 y	6.0-17.0	15-35	5-11	45-76	3-6
2-5 y	5.5-15.5	23-45	5-11	35-65	3-6
5-8 y	5.0-14.5	32-54	5-11	28-48	3-6
13-18 y	4.5-13.0	34-64	5-11	25-45	3-6
Adults	4.5-11.0	35-66	5-11	24-44	3-6

Age	Eosinophils	Basophils	Atypical Lymphs	No. of NRBCs
0-3 d	0-2	0-1	0-8	0-2
1-2 wk	0-2	0-1	0-8	0
1-6 mo	0-3	0-1	0-8	0
7 mo to 2 y	0-3	0-1	0-8	0
2-5 y	0-3	0-1	0-8	0
5-8 y	0-3	0-1	0-8	0
13-18 y	0-3	0-1	0-8	0
Adults	0-3	0-1	0-8	0

Segs = segmented neutrophils   Lymphs = lymphocytes
Bands = band neutrophils   Monos = monocytes

Erythrocyte Sedimentation Rates and Reticulocyte Counts

Sedimentation rate, Westergren	Children	0-20 mm/hour
	Adult male	0-15 mm/hour
	Adult female	0-20 mm/hour
Sedimentation rate, Wintrobe	Children	0-13 mm/hour
	Adult male	0-10 mm/hour
	Adult female	0-15 mm/hour
Reticulocyte count	Newborns	2%-6%
	1-6 mo	0%-2.8%
	Adults	0.5%-1.5%

REFERENCE VALUES FOR CHILDREN

Chemistry

Albumin	0-1 y	2-4 g/dL
	1 y to adult	3.5-5.5 g/dL
Ammonia	Newborns	90-150 µg/dL
	Children	40-120 µg/dL
	Adults	18-54 µg/dL
Amylase	Newborns	0-60 units/L
	Adults	30-110 units/L
Bilirubin, conjugated, direct	Newborns	<1.5 mg/dL
	1 mo to adult	0-0.5 mg/dL
Bilirubin, total	0-3 d	2-10 mg/dL
	1 mo to adult	0-1.5 mg/dL
Bilirubin, unconjugated, indirect		0.6-10.5 mg/dL
Calcium	Newborns	7-12 mg/dL
	0-2 y	8.8-11.2 mg/dL
	2 y to adult	9-11 mg/dL
Calcium, ionized, whole blood		4.4-5.4 mg/dL
Carbon dioxide, total		23-33 mEq/L
Chloride		95-105 mEq/L
Cholesterol	Newborns	45-170 mg/dL
	0-1 y	65-175 mg/dL
	1-20 y	120-230 mg/dL
Creatinine	0-1 y	≤0.6 mg/dL
	1 y to adult	0.5-1.5 mg/dL
Glucose	Newborns	30-90 mg/dL
	0-2 y	60-105 mg/dL
	Children to adults	70-110 mg/dL
Iron	Newborns	110-270 µg/dL
	Infants	30-70 µg/dL
	Children	55-120 µg/dL
	Adults	70-180 µg/dL
Iron binding	Newborns	59-175 µg/dL
	Infants	100-400 µg/dL
	Adults	250-400 µg/dL
Lactic acid, lactate		2-20 mg/dL
Lead, whole blood		<30 µg/dL
Lipase	Children	20-140 units/L
	Adults	0-190 units/L
Magnesium		1.5-2.5 mEq/L
Osmolality, serum		275-296 mOsm/kg
Osmolality, urine		50-1400 mOsm/kg

Chemistry

Phosphorus	Newborns	4.2-9 mg/dL
	6 wk to ≤18 mo	3.8-6.7 mg/dL
	18 mo to 3 y	2.9-5.9 mg/dL
	3-15 y	3.6-5.6 mg/dL
	>15 y	2.5-5 mg/dL
Potassium, plasma	Newborns	4.5-7.2 mEq/L
	2 d to 3 mo	4-6.2 mEq/L
	3 mo to 1 y	3.7-5.6 mEq/L
	1-16 y	3.5-5 mEq/L
Protein, total	0-2 y	4.2-7.4 g/dL
	>2 y	6-8 g/dL
Sodium		136-145 mEq/L
Triglycerides	Infants	0-171 mg/dL
	Children	20-130 mg/dL
	Adults	30-200 mg/dL
Urea nitrogen, blood	0-2 y	4-15 mg/dL
	2 y to adult	5-20 mg/dL
Uric acid	Male	3-7 mg/dL
	Female	2-6 mg/dL

ENZYMES

Alanine aminotransferase (ALT)	0-2 mo	8-78 units/L
(SGPT)	>2 mo	8-36 units/L
Alkaline phosphatase (ALKP)	Newborns	60-130 units/L
	0-16 y	85-400 units/L
	>16 y	30-115 units/L
Aspartate aminotransferase (AST)	Infants	18-74 units/L
(SGOT)	Children	15-46 units/L
	Adults	5-35 units/L
Creatine kinase (CK)	Infants	20-200 units/L
	Children	10-90 units/L
	Adult male	0-206 units/L
	Adult female	0-175 units/L
Lactate dehydrogenase (LDH)	Newborns	290-501 units/L
	1 mo to 2 y	110-144 units/L
	>16 y	60-170 units/L

BLOOD GASES

	Arterial	Capillary	Venous
pH	7.35-7.45	7.35-7.45	7.32-7.42
pCO_2 (mm Hg)	35-45	35-45	38-52
pO_2 (mm Hg)	70-100	60-80	24-48
HCO_3 (mEq/L)	19-25	19-25	19-25
TCO_2 (mEq/L)	19-29	19-29	23-33
O_2 saturation (%)	90-95	90-95	40-70
Base excess (mEq/L)	-5 to +5	-5 to +5	-5 to +5

THYROID FUNCTION TESTS

T_4 (thyroxine)	1-7 d	10.1-20.9 µg/dL
	8-14 d	9.8-16.6 µg/dL
	1 mo to 1 y	5.5-16 µg/dL
	>1 y	4-12 µg/dL
FTI	1-3 d	9.3-26.6
	1-4 wks	7.6-20.8
	1-4 mo	7.4-17.9
	4-12 mo	5.1-14.5
	1-6 y	5.7-13.3
	>6 y	4.8-14
T_3 by RIA	Newborns	100-470 ng/dL
	1-5 y	100-260 ng/dL
	5-10 y	90-240 ng/dL
	10 y to adult	70-210 ng/dL
T_3 uptake		35%-45%
TSH	Cord	3-22 µU/mL
	1-3 d	<40 µU/mL
	3-7 d	<25 µU/mL
	>7 d	0-10 µU/mL

ALPHABETICAL KEY WORD INDEX

ALPHABETICAL KEY WORD INDEX

Z

NOTES

NOTES

NOTES

NOTES

NOTES

NOTES

Other Titles Offered by Lexi-Comp

DRUG INFORMATION HANDBOOK (International edition available)

by Charles Lacy, PharmD; Lora L. Armstrong, BSPharm; Morton P. Goldman, PharmD; and Leonard L. Lance, BSPharm

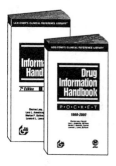

Specifically compiled and designed for the healthcare professional requiring quick access to concisely stated comprehensive data concerning clinical use of medications.

The Drug Information Handbook is an ideal portable drug information resource, containing 1250 drug monographs. Each monograph typically provides the reader with up to 29 key points of data concerning clinical use and dosing of the medication. Material provided in the Appendix section is recognized by many users to be, by itself, well worth the purchase of the handbook.

All medications found in the *Drug Information Handbook*, 7th Edition are included in the abridged Pocket edition.

PEDIATRIC DOSAGE HANDBOOK (International edition available)

by Carol K. Taketomo, PharmD; Jane Hurlburt Hodding, PharmD; and Donna M. Kraus, PharmD

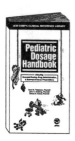

Special considerations must frequently be taken into account when dosing medications for the pediatric patient. This highly regarded quick reference handbook is a compilation of recommended pediatric doses based on current literature as well as the practical experience of the authors and their many colleagues who work every day in the pediatric clinical setting.

The Pediatric Dosage Handbook 6th Edition includes neonatal dosing, drug administration, and extemporaneous preparations for 640 medications used in pediatric medicine.

GERIATRIC DOSAGE HANDBOOK (International edition available)

by Todd P. Semla, PharmD, BCPS, FCCP; Judith L. Beizer, PharmD, FASCP; and Martin D. Higbee, PharmD, CGP

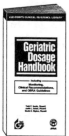

Many physiologic changes occur with aging, some of which affect the pharmacokinetics or pharmacodynamics of medications. Strong consideration should also be given to the effect of decreased renal or hepatic functions in the elderly as well as the probability of the geriatric patient being on multiple drug regimens.

Healthcare professionals working with nursing homes and assisted living facilities will find the 770 drug monographs contained in this handbook to be an invaluable source of helpful information.

To order call toll free: 1-800-837-LEXI (5394)

DRUG INFORMATION HANDBOOK FOR ADVANCED PRACTICE NURSING

by Beatrice B. Turkoski, RN, PhD; Brenda R. Lance, RN, MSN; Mark F. Bonfiglio, PharmD

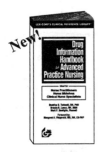

This handbook was designed specifically to meet the needs of Nurse Practitioners, Clinical Nurse Specialists, Nurse Midwives and graduate nursing students. The handbook is a unique resource for detailed, accurate information, which is vital to support the advanced practice nurse's role in patient drug therapy management.

A concise introductory section reviews topics related to Pharmacotherapeutics.

Over 4750 U.S., Canadian, and Mexican medications are covered in the 1055 monographs. Drug data is presented in an easy-to-use, alphabetically organized format covering up to 46 key points of information. Monographs are cross-referenced to an Appendix of over 230 pages of valuable comparison tables and additional information. Also included are two indices, Pharmacologic Category and Controlled Substance, which facilitate comparison between agents.

DRUG INFORMATION HANDBOOK FOR NURSING

by Beatrice B. Turkoski, RN, PhD; Brenda R. Lance, RN, MSN; Mark F. Bonfiglio, PharmD

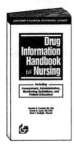

Registered Professional Nurses and upper-division nursing students involved with drug therapy will find this handbook provides quick access to drug data in a concise easy-to-use format.

Over 4750 U.S., Canadian, and Mexican medications are covered with up to 43 key points of information in each monograph. The handbook contains basic pharmacology concepts and nursing issues such as patient factors that influence drug therapy (ie, pregnancy, age, weight, etc) and general nursing issues (ie, assess-ment, administration, monitoring, and patient education). The Appendix contains over 220 pages of valuable information.

DRUG INFORMATION HANDBOOK FOR PHYSICIAN ASSISTANTS

by Michael J. Rudzinski, RPA-C, RPh; J. Fred Bennes, RPA, RPh

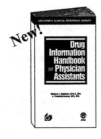

This comprehensive and easy-to-use handbook covers over 3600 drugs and also includes monographs on commonly used herbal products. There are up to 24 key fields of information per monograph, such as Pediatric And Adult Dosing With Adjustments for Renal/hepatic Impairment, Labeled And Unlabeled Uses, Pregnancy & Breast-feeding Precautions, and Special PA issues. Brand (U.S. and Canadian) and generic names are listed alphabetically for rapid access. It is fully cross-referenced by page number and includes alphabetical and pharmacologic indices.

INFECTIOUS DISEASES HANDBOOK

by Carlos M. Isada MD; Bernard L. Kasten Jr. MD; Morton P. Goldman PharmD; Larry D. Gray PhD; and Judith A. Aberg MD

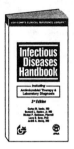

This four-in-one quick reference is concerned with the identification and treatment of infectious diseases. Each of the four sections of the book (166 disease syndromes, 152 organisms, 238 laboratory tests, and 295 antimicrobials) contain related information and cross-referencing to one or more of the other three sections.

The disease syndrome section provides the clinical presentation, differential diagnosis, diagnostic tests, and drug therapy recommended for treatment of more common infectious diseases. The organism section presents the microbiology, epidemiology, diagnosis, and treatment of each organism. The laboratory diagnosis section describes performance of specific tests and procedures. The antimicrobial therapy section presents important facts and considerations regarding each drug recommended for specific diseases of organisms.

ANESTHESIOLOGY & CRITICAL CARE DRUG HANDBOOK

by Andrew J. Donnelly, PharmD; Francesca E. Cunningham, PharmD; and Verna L. Baughman, MD

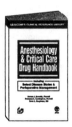

Contains over 512 generic medications with up to 25 fields of information presented in each monograph. It also contains the following Special Issues and Topics: Allergic Reaction, Anesthesia for Cardiac Patients in Noncardiac Surgery, Anesthesia for Obstetric Patients in Nonobstetric Surgery, Anesthesia for Patients With Liver Disease, Chronic Pain Management, Chronic Renal Failure, Conscious Sedation, Perioperative Management of Patients on Antiseizure Medication, Substance Abuse and Anesthesia.

The Appendix includes Abbreviations & Measurements, Anesthesiology Information, Assessment of Liver & Renal Function, Comparative Drug Charts, Infectious Disease-Prophylaxis & Treatment, Laboratory Values, Therapy Recommendation, Toxicology, *and much more . . .*

DRUG INFORMATION HANDBOOK FOR ONCOLOGY

by Dominic A. Solimando, Jr, MA; Linda R. Bressler, PharmD, BCOP; Polly E. Kintzel, PharmD, BCPS, BCOP; Mark C. Geraci, PharmD, BCOP

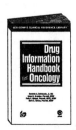

Presented in a concise and uniform format, this book contains the most comprehensive collection of oncology-related drug information available. Organized like a dictionary for ease of use, drugs can be found by looking up the *brand or generic name!*

This book contains 253 monographs, including over 1100 Antineoplastic Agents and Ancillary Medications.

It also contains up to 33 fields of information per monograph including Use, U.S. Investigational, Bone Marrow/Blood Cell Transplantation, Vesicant, Emetic Potential. A Special Topics Section, Appendix, and Therapeutic Category & Key Word Index are valuable features to this book, as well.

To order call toll free: 1-800-837-LEXI (5394)

DRUG-INDUCED NUTRIENT DEPLETION HANDBOOK

by Ross Pelton, RPh, PhD, CCN; James B. LaValle, RPh, DHM, NMD, CCN; Ernest B. Hawkins, RPh, MS; Daniel L. Krinsky, RPh, MS

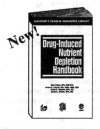

A complete and up-to-date listing of all drugs known to deplete the body of nutritional compounds.

This book is alphabetically organized and provides extensive cross-referencing to related information in the various sections of the book. Nearly 150 generic drugs that cause nutrient depletion are identified and are cross-referenced to more detailed descriptions of the nutrients depleted and their actions. Symptoms of deficiencies, and sources of repletion are also included. This book also contains a Studies and Abstracts section, a valuable Appendix, and Alphabetical & Pharma-cological Indices.

NATURAL THERAPEUTICS POCKET GUIDE

by James B. LaValle, RPh, DHM, NMD, CCN; Daniel L. Krinsky, RPh, MS; Ernest B. Hawkins, RPh, MS; Ross Pelton, RPh, PhD, CCN; Nancy Ashbrook Willis, BA, JD

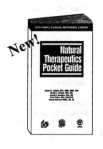

Provides condition-specific information on common uses of natural therapies.

Containing information on over 70 conditions, each including the following: review of condition, decision tree, list of commonly recommended herbals, nutritional supplements, homeopathic remedies, lifestyle modifications, and contraindications & warnings. Provides herbal/nutritional/nutraceutical monographs with over 10 fields including references, reported uses, dosage, pharmacology, toxicity, warnings & interactions, and cautions & contraindications.

Appendix: drug-nutrient depletion, herb-drug interactions, drug-nutrient interaction, herbal medicine use in pediatrics, unsafe herbs, and reference of top herbals.

DRUG INFORMATION HANDBOOK FOR CARDIOLOGY

by Bradley G. Phillips, PharmD; Virend K. Somers, MD, Dphil

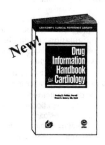

An ideal resource for physicians, pharmacists, nurses, residents, and students. This handbook was designed to provide the most current information on cardio-vascular agents and other ancillary medications.

- Each monograph includes information on Special Cardiovascular Considerations and I.V. to Oral Equivalency
- Alphabetically organized by brand and generic name
- Appendix contains information on Hypertension, Anticoagulation, Cytochrome P-450, Hyperlipidemia, Antiarrhythmia, and Comparative Drug Charts
- Special Topics/Issues include Emerging Risk Factors for Cardiovascular Disease, Treatment of Cardiovas-cular Disease in the Diabetic, Cardiovascular Stress Testing, and Experimental Cardiovascular Therapeutic Strategies in the New Millenium, and much more . . .

DRUG INFORMATION HANDBOOK FOR THE CRIMINAL JUSTICE PROFESSIONAL
by Marcelline Burns, PhD; Thomas E. Page, MA; and Jerrold B. Leikin, MD

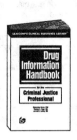

Compiled and designed for police officers, law enforcement officials, and legal professionals who are in need of a reference which relates to information on drugs, chemical substances, and other agents that have abuse and/or impairment potential. This handbook covers over 450 medications, agents, and substances. Each monograph is presented in a consistent format and contains up to 33 fields of information including Scientific Name, Commonly Found In, Abuse Potential, Impairment Potential, Use, When to Admit to Hospital, Mechanism of Toxic Action, Signs & Symptoms of Acute Overdose, Drug Interactions, Warnings/Precautions, and Reference Range. There are many diverse chapter inclusions as well as a glossary of medical terms for the layman along with a slang street drug listing. The Appendix contains Chemical, Bacteriologic, and Radiologic Agents - Effects and Treatment; Controlled Substances - Uses and Effects; Medical Examiner Data; Federal Trafficking Penalties, and much more.

DRUG INFORMATION HANDBOOK FOR PSYCHIATRY
(International edition available) by Matthew A. Fuller, PharmD; Martha Sajatovic, MD

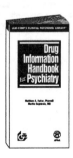

As a source for comprehensive and clinically relevant drug information for the mental health professional, this handbook is alphabetically arranged by generic and brand name for ease-of-use. It covers over 4,000 brand names and up to 32 key fields of information including effect on mental status and effect on psychiatric treatment.

A special topics/issues section includes psychiatric assessment, overview of selected major psychiatric disorders, clinical issues in the use of major classes of psychotropic medications, psychiatric emergencies, special populations, diagnostic and statistical manual of mental disorders (DSM-IV), and suggested readings. Also contains a valuable Appendix section, as well as, a Therapeutic Category Index and an Alphabetical Index.

LABORATORY TEST HANDBOOK CONCISE version
by David S. Jacobs MD, FACP; Wayne R. DeMott, MD, FACP; Harold J. Grady, PhD; Rebecca T. Horvat, PhD; Douglas W. Huestis, MD; and Bernard L. Kasten Jr., MD, FACP

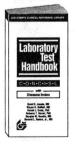

The authors of Lexi-Comp's highly regarded Laboratory Test Handbook, 4th Edition have selected and extracted key information for presentation in this portable abridged version.

The Laboratory Test Handbook Concise contains more than 800 tests entries for quick reference and is ideal for residents, nurses, and medical students or technologists requiring information concerning patient preparation, specimen collection and handling, and test result interpretation.

DRUG INFORMATION HANDBOOK FOR DENTISTRY

by Richard L. Wynn, BSPharm, PhD; Timothy F. Meiller, DDS, PhD; and Harold L. Crossley, DDS, PhD

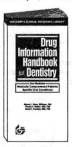

This handbook presents dental management and therapeutic considerations in medically compromised patients. Issues covered include oral manifestations of drugs, pertinent dental drug interactions, and dosing of drugs in dental treatment.

Selected oral medicine topics requiring therapeutic intervention include managing the patient with acute or chronic pain including TMD, managing the patient with oral bacterial or fungal infections, current therapeutics in periodontal patients, managing the patient receiving chemotherapy or radiation for the treatment of cancer, managing the anxious patient, managing dental office emergencies, and treatment of common oral lesions.

DENTAL OFFICE MEDICAL EMERGENCIES

by Timothy F. Meiller, DDS, PhD; Richard L. Wynn, BSPharm, PhD; Ann Marie McMullin, MD; Cynthia Biron, RDH, EMT, MA; Harold L. Crossley, DDS, PhD

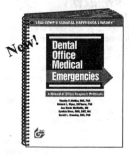

Designed specifically for general dentists during times of emergency. A tabbed paging system allows for quick access to specific crisis events. Created with urgency in mind, it is spiral bound and drilled with a hole for hanging purposes.

- Basic Action Plan for Stabilization
- Loss of Consciousness / Respiratory Distress / Chest Pain
- Allergic / Drug Reactions
- Altered Sensation / Changes in Affect
- Management of Acute Bleeding
- Office Preparedness / Procedures and Protocols

DIAGNOSTIC PROCEDURE HANDBOOK

by Joseph A. Golish, MD

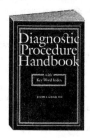

An ideal companion to the Laboratory Test Handbook this publication details 295 diagnostic procedures including Allergy, Immunology/Rheumotology, Infectious Disease, Cardiology, Critical Care, Gastroenterology, Nephrology, Urology, Hematology, Neurology, Ophthalmology, Pulmonary Function, Pulmonary Medicine, Computed Tomography, Diagnostic Radiology, Invasive Radiology, Magnetic Resonance Imaging, Nuclear Medicine, and Ultrasound. A great reference handbook for healthcare professionals at any level of training and experience.

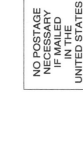

LEXI-COMP, INC

1100 Terex Road · Hudson, OH 44236

BUSINESS REPLY MAIL

FIRST-CLASS MAIL   PERMIT NO 689   HUDSON, OH

POSTAGE WILL BE PAID BY ADDRESSEE

LEXI-COMP, INC.
Clinician's Endodontic Handbook
1100 Terex Road
Hudson, OH 44236-9915

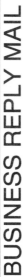

Thank you!

for purchasing Lexi-Comp's *Clinician's Endodontic Handbook*

Return this postage-paid card so we can keep you up-to-date on all the latest products, promotions and upgrades.

☐ Please put me on your **"Mailing List".**

☐ Please put me on your **"Standing Order List"** to automatically receive the new edition each year.

Please print the title of the book here that you would like to receive a new edition of automatically each year.

☐ Please send me information on **quantity discounts.**

Name (First): _____ (Last): _____

Title / Occupation: _____

Institution / Company: _____

Address: _____

City: _____ State/Province: _____

Zip/Postal Code: _____ Country: _____

Telephone: (___) _____ Fax: (___) _____

E-Mail Address: _____

OTHER AREAS OF INTEREST (listed alphabetically by topic):

☐ Advanced Practice Nursing Drug Information   ☐ Geriatric Dosage Information

☐ Allied Health Professional Drug Information   ☐ Infectious Diseases

☐ Anesthesiology & Critical Care Drug Information   ☐ Laboratory Tests

☐ Cardiology Drug Information   ☐ Natural Therapeutics

☐ Clinician's Endodontic Handbook   ☐ Nursing Drug Information

☐ Criminal Justice Professional Drug Information   ☐ Oncology Drug Information

☐ Dental Office Medical Emergencies   ☐ Pediatric Dosage

☐ Dentistry Drug Information   ☐ PA's Drug Information

☐ Diagnostic Procedures   ☐ Poisoning & Toxicology

☐ Drug-Induced Nutrient Depletion   ☐ Psychiatry Drug Information

☐ Drug Information   ☐ Psychotropic Drug Information

ALSO INTERESTED IN THE FOLLOWING:

☐ Formulary or Laboratory Custom Publishing Service

☐ Lexi-Comp's CRL™ on CD-ROM   ___ Academic ___ Personal ___ Institutional

☐ Lexi-Comp database on a hand-held device ___ Palm Pilot ___ Windows CE™ ___ Other